Frontiers of Health

Frontiers of Health
From Healing to Wholeness

Dr CHRISTINE R. PAGE
MB, BS, MRCGP, DCH, DRCOG, MFHom

SAFFRON WALDEN
THE C.W. DANIEL COMPANY LIMITED

DEDICATION

I would like to thank my mother,
Pat Jarvis and the many patients
who were my teachers.

First published in Great Britain in 1992
by The C.W. Daniel Company Limited
1 Church Path, Saffron Walden
Essex, CB10 1JP, England

ISBN 0 85207 256 2

Revised edition 1994

This book has been printed on part-recycled paper

Designed and Produced in association with
Book Production Consultants, Cambridge
Typeset by Cambridge Photosetting Services
Printed in England by St Edmundsbury Press Limited,
Bury St Edmunds, Suffolk

CONTENTS

INTRODUCTION

One of the questions I am often asked is: "when did you first become interested in spiritual matters?"

My answer is that I do not remember a time when I was not aware of the spiritual world.

My mother was involved in spiritual healing and I recall listening to her as she talked about "fringe medicine" and recounted esoteric teachings. For me she was reinforcing views that were already part of my own inner truth.

Little did I imagine how important this early introduction to the links between the mind, the body and the spirit would be in my later life and especially in my chosen career.

My earliest childhood memory is when I was about 14 months old. I remember watching as one of my favourite dolls fell between two wooden chairs and smashed into tiny pieces. I was devastated; I watched with horror as the pieces were unceremoniously resigned to the dustbin. I could not believe that it was not possible to make this life, however imaginary, whole again and that so little was done in pursuit of this goal.

That incident appears to have triggered an inner desire to do all in my power to help people towards health and wholeness. In fact, the words health and healing come from the Germanic word "wholeness" or to make whole. I soon realised that such healing had to start with the helper, myself.

When it came to the time to make a decision concerning a career, I chose one of the health professions with the hope that here I would be in a position to help people along their path in life, hopefully with a caring but objective approach.

So when I entered the doors of my medical school some 18 years ago I was full of hope that here was the fulfilment of a dream. On my first day, with eight fellow students, I stood around a table upon which lay my first dead body ready to learn all I could about a human being.

It soon dawned that there was only one problem, this body was missing an essential item ... life itself.

I therefore eagerly awaited my graduation onto the wards. Here we, as medical students, were licensed to poke and prod any poor unsuspecting patient in order to expand our knowledge of the disease state. Any verbal interruption from the patient was often seen as an unwelcome intrusion.

"Just answer my questions, please". There was little time for discussions of social and emotional problems.

I recognise from my own career that, when working in a hospital, it is often difficult to remember that all patients have another life outside and that, first and foremost, they are people.

As I listened to my patients talk it became clear that many of them had stressful lives including marriage breakdowns, problems with the children, job losses, sick relatives, etc. and that despite my medical training I was inadequately prepared to deal with such problems.

Diseases of the body and the mind were definitely seen as separate entities, with the latter referred to the psychology or psychiatry departments of the hospital. Any connections which were made came under the title of psychosomatic illness (psyche- mind, soma- body).

However, it was often the case that this term was used as a diagnosis when extensive tests had failed to reveal a cause for the patient's illness. The patient left the doctor's surgery with the belief that their symptoms were "all in their mind" which created further stress and a feeling of hopelessness.

It became obvious that this was a major flaw in the healing package offered by the medical profession, one which thankfully is now being addressed in modern medical training.

During this time I was having my own problems. The experience of being in close proximity to the suffering of others caused havoc with my sensitivity. I was overwhelmed by the physical and emotional pain of my patients and felt that I was not in a position to offer aid due to lack of knowledge.

As a result, on several occasions, I slid gracefully to the ground in a dead faint at the sight of blood and pain. The solution at that time was to bury my feelings behind a frenzy of activity whenever I felt vaguely inadequate.

The donning of a white coat added extra protection to a sensitive soul. Within it I became anonymous and appeared detached, unemotional and professional. Or so I believed.

In retrospect I see that all I achieved was to bury my feelings and I believe that for many doctors this approach causes a great deal of harm and should be looked upon as one of the commonest causes of our high suicide and alcoholism rates.

It took some time to realise how important it was to value myself for just "being there" and that although my medical expertise was important, it was unconditional compassion which enhanced the healing process.

During my studies I became more and more aware that, despite a similar diagnosis, different patients reacted in different ways to the disease and to the chosen treatment.

There was no such thing as a "sure bet" as to whether a patient would leave the hospital fully cured or would die without any advance warning.

I was trained to talk in terms of statistical prognosis. "80% of people die with a certain disease within 2 years".

Nobody ever told me what happened to the other 20%.

What made them live? Why were they different?

I concluded that not all disease could be attributed to the germ. There have been numerous studies which have shown that despite the existence of a virus or bacteria within a close community, or where on several occasions these were administered in error to a group of individuals, only a small proportion of those involved developed symptoms of disease.

In the nineteenth century Claude Bernard, a great medical researcher, wrote: "Illnesses hover constantly about us, their seeds blown by the wind, but they do not set into the terrain unless the terrain is ready to receive them".

Pasteur, the father of microbiology, is reputed to have said on his deathbed: "Bernard is right. The germ is nothing; the terrain is all".

The terrain equates to the environment and this must include both our inner and outer worlds.

Further evidence revealed that non-identical twins brought up in the same environment showed wide variations in their personality and in the diseases which they acquired throughout their lives. Similarly, not all smokers died of heart or lung disease, not all drinkers had liver damage and the same stress factors did not affect all people in the same way.

The variations within disease patterns must come from within and, with this in mind, I focussed my attention on the other factors involved in the holistic paradigm ... the mind and the spirit.

In the 70s, it became fashionable to talk about stress. It was seen as a widespread problem affecting people of all ages and in all walks of life and became an acceptable answer in the search for the cause of many chronic diseases.

But although stress could be identified as a problem, it appeared more difficult to eradicate despite attempts to relax, meditate, etc.

I concluded that it was not the stress which was the problem but the strain which we felt when it was applied.

Stress is a fundamental requirement for life. In the dictionary it is defined as "... an impelling force applied to a form or structure". The word impelling not only signifies forward movement but also the degree of importance placed upon such an action. Without this we would vegetate, fail to grow and die of lack of primary nourishment.

Strain is defined as "... to be stretched tight beyond the legitimate range". Strain is registered when we move beyond our optimal range of existence, forced on by emotional pressures such as fear and guilt. I believe that such influences are the primary cause of many diseases.

The effects of strain are commonly seen in the physical body as in the case when an extremely heavy load is lifted from the ground resulting in a slipped disc. When we take on too much work in the office the strain may manifest in the form of irritability or weeping, or manifest in the physical body as a headache.

Whatever the signs or symptoms whether physical or mental, the answer is the same; reduce the amount of stretch to within the normal range and the signs of dis-stress will disappear.

The only problem here is that it appears there is no "normal range" for the whole human race or even for members of the same family or same age group.

Appley and Trumbull, who were stress researchers in 1967, concluded that reaction to stress varies considerably from individual to individual and from response to response.

The individual may in fact react to the same stressor in a different manner at different presentations.

In my quest for understanding the connection between the mind and the body, I came across the studies carried out by Greer, et al (1979), who recognised four categories of coping mechanisms adopted by patients with breast cancer. Most patients exhibit more than one of these mechanisms during their illness, but there is usually one which is prominent. These are:

a) **Stoic acceptance;** here there is a realistic appreciation of the facts of the illness which is shown by a calm, fatalistic and a rather passive attitude towards the disease.

This is the commonest attitude adopted and connects closely with personality traits which are often found in those who develop cancer.

b) **Helplessness/hopelessness;** despair about the illness and no motivation to adapt.

This is the closest to a state of depression and is commonly seen at the beginning of any grieving process.

c) **Fighting spirit;** here the patient is determined to fight their illness and to recover from it.

These individuals have probably always been fighters and have a desire to be in control of any situation especially their own treatment. They will read all the books, seek second opinions and organise support groups.

d) **Denial;** the failure to absorb the knowledge concerning the diagnosis and its implications.

There is an apparent amnesia covering any aspects of the disease especially those connected with the diagnosis and therefore a failure to ask appropriate questions when time is given for such an exchange.

In the case of denial, an observer who personally prefers the honest approach will see the patient's refusal to talk about his or her cancer as a challenge. They will take it upon themselves to encourage the patient to talk about their fears and concerns in order to prevent the suppression of emotions they believe may lead to further disabling problems.

As I learnt to my cost, such an approach has little regard for the wishes of the patient and is purely satisfying the ego of the observer.

Having been presented with the truth clearly and simply, the patient has every right to choose not to talk about the subject which manifests as a denial.

I remember my own naivety when faced with a patient who was dying of lung cancer. When I entered the house, I was met by the wife, who hurried me past the patient and into the kitchen where I was told in great detail about her husband's cancer and the present problems.

We then went back into the bedroom where the husband lay and started to talk about the weather and the minor problems of the illness.

After another similar visit, I asked the wife whether her husband was aware of the diagnosis and if he realised he was extremely ill. She said that she was not sure because they never talked about his ill health.

Being a good conscientious doctor, I felt that the truth should be brought into the open and went back into the bedroom.

"Do you know what is wrong with you?" I asked.

"Yes, I have cancer" he replied.

"Do you know how ill you are?" I continued.

"Yes, I know I am dying".

"Have you talked to your wife about this?" I asked.

"No, I do not want to worry her" he replied.

As I left the house his wife said with a sigh:

"So he knows, and there is no use in pretending anymore."

Seeing her face I realised I had betrayed their trust in me and acted against the wishes of the couple in my misplaced desire to help.

The next day the patient's condition deteriorated and he went into hospital.

He did manage to come home for a brief period before he died and I felt that it was appropriate that I was called to see him in his dying moments, and that I could be there to comfort his wife in the days that followed.

My wish to bring everything into the open had destroyed the delicate fabric of denial which had been built up between these two people as a coping mechanism. As with many experiences within my working life, I felt very humbled, but grateful to learn such an important lesson from my patients.

Coping mechanisms are used not only in cases of cancer but within any situation when there is change in the flow of life. Doctors use these mechanisms every day to deal with the stresses which they encounter, especially those which affect them deeply.

Lessons concerned with the emotional aspects of dying, death and grieving were not part of my medical training. At the age of 23 years and without formal tuition, I was expected to know how to tell someone that they or their relative were dying. I questioned this omission from the syllabus and came to the conclusion that the reason why it was not taught was because many people, including those in the medical professions, have not come to terms with their own mortality.

I had first-hand experience at an early age of watching someone I loved die, and dealing with the subsequent grief. Fortunately, most people do not have to face this situation until they are much older. And yet they are asked to give advice and support in such matters when their training is so inadequate. I feel strongly that this is another area which should no longer be relegated to the realms of religion but be encompassed in medical training. I would like to believe that this indeed has happened and that the modern houseman is more equipped to deal with such important issues.

There is no right or wrong way to deal with a problem and all those within the caring professions should recognise that they are not there to judge but rather to give guidance and support where appropriate.

Unfortunately, it is not always so easy to be non-judgemental due to the practitioner's own human frailties. This is compounded by the position of authority given by society to those in the caring professions.

The opinion of the doctor, and the way in which it is presented, is seen to influence greatly the patient's disease process as shown by studies on the placebo effect.

Positive reinforcement, the placebo, given by the doctor whilst prescribing a treatment is estimated to relieve symptoms in 30% of patients. This has been verified in research studies where the reinforcement was given alongside a sugar tablet which secretly replaced the real drug.

Deepak Chopra in his book Quantum Healing (1989) talks about the "Nocebo" effect which is the negative placebo response. This is a situation where patients are given negative information which leads to a deterioration of their condition.

"You won't last the year" or "You'll probably develop side effects of nausea and vomiting with this drug".

Bernie Siegel, in "Love, Medicine and Miracles", tells the story of two men who by mistake were given the wrong diagnosis. The one who had cancer, and statistically should have died, left the hospital: the other, with a minor problem, left the ward in a coffin.

The response of the nocebo effect on the disease state has not been analysed statistically but I would be surprised if it did not equal that of the placebo response.

I have no doubt as to the influence of the mind in the creation and continuation of the disease process and that it does not always need to be negative. For example, it has been observed on oncology wards that when patients are given positive but honest advice concerning the side effects of the drugs, fewer problems actually manifest.

I remember an old woman who "had turned her head to the wall and decided to die". She refused food and drink and was slowly fading. As is common practice in cases of near death, her nephew as next of kin was contacted.

Without any signs of emotion or concern, he calmly asked what time he should visit to collect her belongings and the death certificate. The nurse appalled by his callousness went to inform the aunt that she had spoken to the nephew, omitting certain sections of the conversation.

The aunt hearing what she wanted to hear, ie. that someone in her family cared, immediately turned and asked for something to drink. Consequently, when the nephew arrived to pick up the death certificate, he found his aunt sitting up in bed full of life and vigour.

Matters of life and death are not in the hands of doctors and health practitioners but in the hands of some far greater power. That which is consciously perceived is but the tip of the iceberg. Anybody who attempts to estimate the quantity or quality of life belonging to another person is attempting to play God and is bound to fail along the way.

Amazing things happen when people are ill. They develop strengths which up to that point had been well and truly hidden.

One of the criticisms levelled at me when I speak to groups of doctors is that it is wrong to give false hope and that patients should face up to their morbidity and mortality.

I do not think that we are talking about hope, false or otherwise, but about honesty and truth. We are being asked to give advice on the basis of our years of experience and learning but in the end the decision is that of the patient.

As a newly qualified doctor I believed that I had the answer to all medical problems. As I grew older and wiser I learnt to say "I do not know" adding, where appropriate, "but I know someone who can help".

As doctors I think we believe we are responsible not only for the patient but also for the presence or absence of disease. Such a belief is not limited to the medical profession but can be found within all those who care for the health of others.

My experience is that patients do not ask us to be responsible for their disease, but to care for them in whatever way we decide has the maximum chance of giving peace from suffering which, ultimately, may be to allow the soul to rest.

My training taught me that life was sacrosanct and that death was failure. I believe that while we still view the body and the mind as the totality of the human being we will always fail, for the only certainty of life is that we will all die some day. Life is terminal.

The spirit must be included in any discussion or teaching concerning man and can no longer be relegated to the religious sections of our community.

The failure to address the issues concerning the whole person became more and more apparent in my own work within general practice where I became aware that 80% of my patients had chronic diseases for which I prescribed medicines which, although relieving the symptoms, did not necessarily alter the underlying disease state.

We appeared to be no closer to understanding the riddle of disease than we were 100 years ago despite modern technology. We still did not know why some people died young while others lived to a ripe old age or why some people contracted illness while others remained apparently healthy.

In the search for answers, my attention once again moved to fringe or rather complementary medicine as it was now known.

I saw that in most of these therapies there was an underlying belief in the connection between the mind, the body and the spirit and that many methods such as reflexology, acupuncture and homoeopathy worked with the principle of an energy or life force flowing through the body which in disease had become blocked creating disharmony within the physical form.

To release the block and allow the recreation of harmony was the main aim of most practitioners who worked within these healing arts.

At last I felt I was connecting with my own inner truth that unless we treat the whole person we cannot hope to achieve a cure.

But, despite my involvement in both orthodox and complementary medicine, I still felt that I had little understanding of the meaning of life and how illness fitted into this process. I believed that nothing happened by chance or without a purpose on some level and that illness was no exception.

The significance of disease varies according to the culture in which it is found. In many cultures it is seen as a weakness and equates to failure.

Several of my male patients confess that they would rather die than face the humiliation of admitting that they were ill. Many of them achieve their ambition long before retirement age!

The early doctors understood the importance of the holistic approach. Hippocrates (420BC), the father of modern medicine was trained as a priest healer. These healers were followers of Aesculapius, the Greek god of healing, whose symbol, the single snake around a rod, is still used by many medical institutions. The priest healers believed that total healing must include the mind, the body and the spirit.

In his later life, Hippocrates transferred his allegiance from a holistic view to one which was more reductionist. He stated that he believed the cause of an illness existed purely within the soil of the disease, ie. the physical body. Slowly, this theme was adopted by all those who cared for the sick, and disease was divided into that dealt with by the doctor, that by the priest and that by the psychiatrist.

However, it is interesting to note that until recently every doctor had to take the Hippocratic oath (circa 420BC) which starts:

"I swear by Apollo the physician, by Aesculapius etc.".

As my studies continued, I searched my medical books for reference to the spirit. When none was found, I transferred my attentions to the esoteric teachings which I had met as a child.

I was enthralled by the wisdom within the Alice Bailey books and attended workshops and lectures. Much that I heard struck a chord deep inside and I began to expand my understanding as to the purpose of life on earth.

I believe that we all originate from the one Source which has many names: the Light, God or the Creator. This Source gives birth to many individual lights or souls and each one of us possesses such a soul.

The purpose of our life upon this earth is to develop self-consciousness which means to know and accept ourselves as spiritual beings. As this awareness increases we work towards wholeness and such wholeness brings the ultimate goal, unity with the Creator.

The soul's path on earth provides many experiences which can lead to such growth. In this world of duality we learn to accept and love both our so called negative aspects and our positive aspects for they are all part of the whole.

In order that the soul can work within the earth, it takes on three items of "clothing"; the emotions, the logical mind and the physical body. These three together constitute the personality or ego.

The soul or Self is still firmly linked with the Source of life via the spirit. Through this connection we are aware of ourselves not only as a personality but also as part of the Universal pattern of life.

The soul is not an alien force which is trying to influence us beyond our will but can be seen as a loving parent showing the way to an often fearful child. The soul needs the personality and they need to work together as friends.

One aspect of this life which to some is seen as a gift and to others as a hindrance ... is the presence of freewill.

Freewill equates with choice; choice to accept the experience and choice to learn the lesson which it offers.

For many freewill brings fear of failure and of making a mistake. In truth, there is no such thing as a mistake; nothing is wasted. The most negative events offer some learning for the soul even if it is only not to follow that path again.

Others become lost in the experience and fail to see that it is not the details of the situation which matter but the opportunity for change which is offered.

And what does the Soul want from life?

As I travel the world giving workshops and seeing patients on a one-to-one basis, I am amazed to find that despite the wide variation of cultures, religions and levels of wealth there is always a common theme:

"I want to be myself".

The Self that they talk about contains seven spiritual aspects:

- Self-knowledge
- Self-responsibility
- Self-expression
- Self-love
- Self-worth
- Self-respect
- Self-awareness

Total Self-consciousness encapsulates all these aspects and is a harmonic existence created through unification of the many parts which constitute spiritual man.

For many of us the personality holds sway over the control of our daily life. As the influence shifts from the personality to the soul, this is registered as disharmony by the mind, for it is now receiving the two different vibrations, one being transmitted from the level of the soul and one from the level of the personality.

If the vibration of the soul is simply allowed to replace that of the personality then the shift occurs with minimal disruption to the life of the individual.

However, if there is resistance to change, then initially this disharmony is felt within the mind leading to symptoms of strain; frustration, anger, depression etc. If, despite these messages, no action is taken to change the vibration, then the disharmony can manifest as physical disease.

Such a manifestation not only increases the awareness of the individual to the fact that there is disharmony present (seeing is believing) but also in many cases acts as the vehicle for the change to take place. I believe that this is the process which is occurring in at least 80% of mental and physical disease seen today, which include trauma.

This book is designed to go within; to attempt to make a link between the ancient esoteric knowledge and modern man. Following my years of medical practice I am convinced that to relegate signs and symptoms purely to the means of naming a disease is to ignore a vital clue given to us by the soul itself.

I believe that if we can decode the message of the disease, we can come to a greater understanding as to the area of soul growth being developed at that time.

In this way, we in the caring professions would then be able to support the patient in a more constructive manner and the patient would be able to contribute actively to their healing process.

To have a conscious understanding of the process of soul growth is not essential for life, but I am sure that it makes the journey much easier.

I fully accept the valuable contribution of modern medicine

to health care especially in acute situations. One of my prime tasks is to teach complementary practitioners to know when to refer to orthodox medicine in accordance with the threat posed by the condition to the life force of the patient.

However, true care must include the activities of the mind and the soul. The physical body is purely a vehicle for the soul and the spirit. Treating one aspect in isolation from the others will lead to an incomplete cure although on a physical level the patient may appear healed.

Healing can never restore anybody to their original form.

Disease by its very essence must bring about change in the individual and this point is often misunderstood and even avoided both by the patient and by their practitioner.

My patients often say: "Just make me feel better physically and then I can cope with the emotional problems".

But this is completely the wrong way round. Yes, by relieving the pain and other acute symptoms, the patient is able to have the strength to move forward. But in many cases, until the emotional issues are resolved, disharmony will remain even though the signs of disease can be suppressed by modern drugs.

Once true harmony has been achieved it can never be destroyed. It may be mislaid from time to time but, like riding a bicycle, we never forget the technique once it is learnt.

For true health and wholeness, time is irrelevant. Many people are in such a hurry to restore health that they miss golden opportunities for soul growth. Because of this, the lesson is repeated unnecessarily, until the deeper message of disease is understood.

Others give up and accept their illness not in a positive fashion but with resignation. They "suffer" from a disease ... the word amplifying their feelings.

Both groups have entered a cul-de-sac where there appears to be no way out. I ask that the reader may consider my ideas as a possible means of breaking the deadlock.

In the end it is not relevant what disease is present, what type of personality you are, what astrological sign you were born under or what type of constitution is present.

What is relevant is how you deal with the situations which

come towards you and to use these experiences to enrich and expand soul consciousness.

The material for the book comes from experiences within my own life especially those involved with disease and healing. The names and certain features of the individuals described in the following chapters have been altered to maintain confidentiality. The essence of the story is the same.

Much of the esoteric knowledge comes from the teachings of Alice Bailey who received the information from a Tibetan Master. But in the end it is not the knowledge which is important, but the application of this knowledge to life.

Knowledge is powerless without wisdom and love. If the words which you read strike a chord somewhere and provide understanding to an inner problem then I am well pleased.

If they don't ... then that's fine too.

Chapter 1

The Origin of the Soul

In order to understand the mind, body, spirit connection, I feel that it is necessary to attempt to provide an esoteric explanation behind the origin of spiritual man.

In the world of science the theory of the "Big Bang" is offered as a credible explanation behind the creation of the Universe.

As a parallel in esoteric terms, we learn about an Energy or Divine Life which is the source of all that is visible and invisible within the Universe. Everything in existence is an expression of this One Life.

When this Divine Energy Source takes form, two poles of expression are created which result in the duality of life which is exhibited throughout the universe.

These two aspects of duality are usually described as:

    a) Spirit or the Father.

    b) Matter or the Mother.

Born out of the union between the Father and the Mother is the Son or the Soul.

In view of the fact that the Soul represents the unity between Spirit and Matter it can also been seen that ultimately the Soul is a reflection of the initial Life Energy.

> Out of the One comes the Two.
> Out of Two comes the Three.
> Together they represent the One.

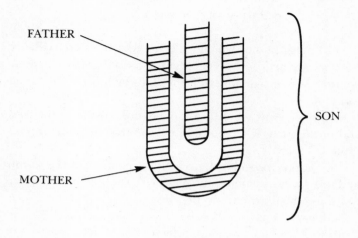

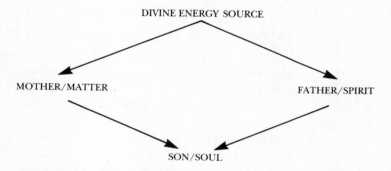

The essence of the Father and Mother express different aspects of Divine Intelligence.

The essence of the Father or Spirit is seen in terms of positivity, masculinity, dominance, outward movement, logic and assertiveness. It expresses the Will to create and with this to grow.

The essence of the Mother or Matter is seen in terms of negativity, femininity, receptiveness, inward movement, sensitivity and nurturing. It expresses the Wisdom to bring together all that is required to nurture the seed of the creator leading to new birth and the continuation of life.

Their union is brought about by the power of attraction or love which manifests as the essence of the Son or Soul.

> Love unites all, leading to the
> extinction of separation.

The energy of the Will is an electrical force whereas that of Love is a magnetic force. Together they create electromagnetic energy which is symbolised by the sun which brings life to all form.

In human terms, we see the father as the provider of the seed and of the materials required in order that the baby should grow.

The mother provides the receptive qualities of the womb and with her wisdom uses the materials provided by the father to gain optimal benefit for the baby.

Both have equal importance in the creation of this child (the Soul) which is an expression of the power of their love.

THE PATH OF THE SOUL

Every living object is created through the interaction between the spirit and matter. Therefore every living object has a soul, from an atom to a planet. In many cases the soul is collective, ie. the same soul for a group of objects.

In man, the soul is individualised creating diversity within an apparently common form.

In the human body, this uniqueness is expressed within the pattern of fingerprints and in the genetic information stored within the chromosomes.

Both spirit and matter contain an innate level of "intelligence" passed down from the original Divine Intelligence. Through their union, the soul is produced which can be seen as the level of consciousness or awareness which is achieved when these two aspects of intelligence meet (Conscious from the Latin -scire; to know).

Such consciousness will depend upon the degree of interaction which takes place between these two aspects and the nature of the form which is expressed.

The various life-forms which inhabit the Earth are expressing

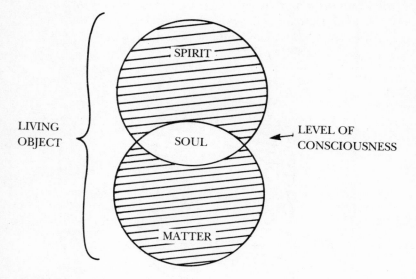

different stages in the development of this consciousness, ie. that of a cell will differ from that of a plant; while some individuals are more spiritually aware than others.

The purpose of life is to increase the level of consciousness through the interaction between spirit and matter until ultimately there is no separation between these two aspects of polarity and the consciousness of the soul and the source become one.

An Analogy

If the spirit were a lighted candle and matter was a piece of ice, it would initially be difficult to see the flame through the ice.

If the ice is brought closer to the flame, it starts to melt and now the light of the flame can be seen more clearly through the water, ie. the water is transmitting the light of the candle.

If the heat of the flame continues to be concentrated upon the water, evaporation will occur until the water is no longer visible and is now fully transmitting the light of the candle.

In conclusion, heat increases the vibrational rate of the molecules of the water, changing it from a solid form, ice, into something far freer and lighter. At the same time it allows easier transmission of the light through the medium of steam.

In a similar manner, harmony is achieved between spirit and matter and is seen to be mutually beneficial to both.

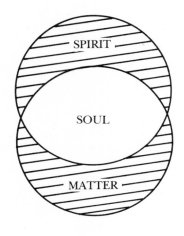

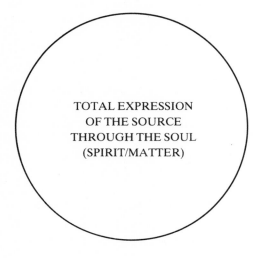

THE PATH OF MAN

Man's journey is to become self-aware or self-conscious … to know himself.

This does not happen overnight but is an evolving process.

He has the capability to see himself as a separate entity from his physical body, his emotions and from his thoughts, ie. separate from his personality which is the collective name for these three aspects of man.

ie.

Man is not his physical world …
his house, his car, his job.
Man is not his emotions … his
anger, his sadness, his fears.
Man is not his thoughts … his
analysis, his knowledge.
Man is not his personality.

This recognition can only come from an objective viewpoint which is identified as the position of the soul of the individual.

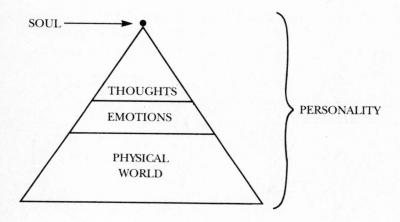

As this awareness grows there is an increase in the conscious appreciation of the spiritual world and man's small but important role in the greater plan.

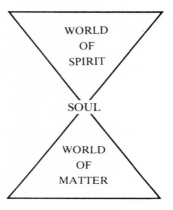

However, the very awareness of the separation between the soul and the personality has created two further poles of existence which need to be united before man can be called a truly spiritual being.

Harmony is created through unity.

Therefore once the individual has reached a level of awareness which recognises the soul as separate from the personality, the energy of the soul, which is linked to that of spirit, must

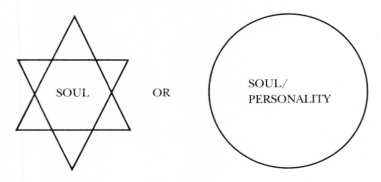

then be brought back down through the thoughts, the emotions and the physical body so that the will of the soul and the personality can become one.

Only then, in esoteric terms, when the soul is fully incarnate in the physical form, can the serpent who dwells at the base of the spine rise up. This is also known as the raising of the Kundalini. Such an action cannot be forced but is a natural result of attaining the necessary steps in the evolution of consciousness.

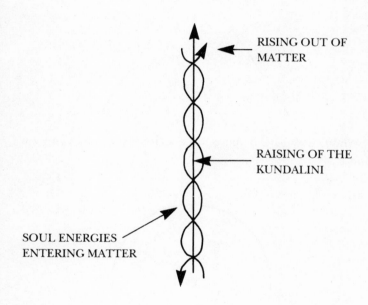

RISING OUT OF
MATTER

RAISING OF THE
KUNDALINI

SOUL ENERGIES
ENTERING MATTER

THE ESSENCE OF DUALITY

The creation of the two poles of existence, spirit and matter and their unification through the formation of the son or the soul is the basis of all life situations.

To experience, to recognise and to accept both poles brings

an awareness that there is no separation but only different expressions of a common principle. All are part of the Greater Creative Energy.

An Analogy

If I view a tepee from the front it appears as a structure with two sides and a central support.

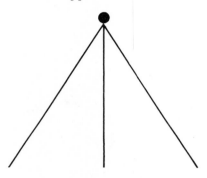

When viewed from above, I see a circle around a common point.

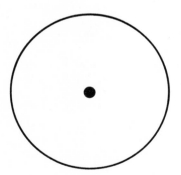

The Chinese Teachings

The concept of duality is also seen in Chinese Philosophy where two opposing but complementary forces called **yin and yang** are described. They express the way in which things function in relation to each other and are used to explain the continual and natural process of change.

Neither can exist without the other; there are no absolutes. We cannot know night unless we know day; we talk about inspiration because we recognise expiration.

Both contain the potential for transformation into the opposite force.

Yin is described as cold, rest, passivity, darkness, responsive, inward and decreasing.

Yang is described as heat, movement, activity, brightness, stimulation, outward and increasing.

The concept of yin and yang is depicted in the Chinese Taoist symbol shown below.

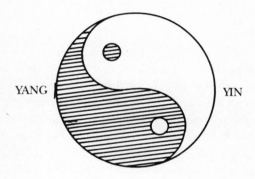

The dividing line shows that the two aspects are always merging. The small contrasting circles show the potential for transformation.

The twists in the movement of a snake or the turns in a spiral also reflect this concept of balance achieved through the unification of two poles of existence.

Chinese philosophy shows that it is impossible to stay in one aspect and ignore the other.

The same concept is revealed within esoteric teachings which speak about the **Universal Law of Balance and Equilibrium**. This states that if one aspect of polarity is expressed in

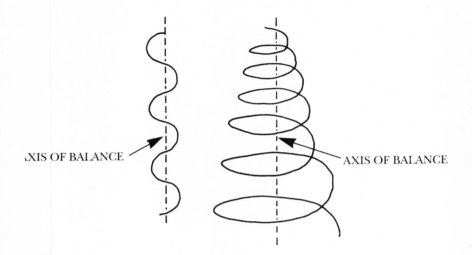

AXIS OF BALANCE   AXIS OF BALANCE

an extreme state then its complementary aspect must subsequently be expressed to re-balance the situation.

Much of disease is an attempt to correct an imbalance through the medium of the physical form. It is an inevitability for, according to the above law, harmony needs to be re-established.

Therefore any apparent breakdown on the part of the physical or mental body should be seen as the action of a friend rather than that of an enemy.

Breakdown is to break out.

Disease is not a punishment or a sign of weakness but a natural process in the recreation of equilibrium.

For example
A business man who continues to burn the candle at both ends with an excess intake of alcohol, spices and coffee may manifest an illness which will curb his excesses, such as, an ulcer or something which will slow him down, a heart attack. To the business man they may be viewed as an inconvenience … to spiritual man they are seen as his salvation.

Ignore the need for change and more permanent ways are presented in order to redress the imbalance.

Many states of ill-health are brought about by a failure to let go of old thoughts, attitudes, emotions and possessions which leads to an extreme expression of one aspect.

Fear and guilt are the commonest reasons given for the need to hold onto the past or to fail to move forward into the future. To release these old friends requires faith and this can only come when we are in touch with our own inner being.

However, blind faith, such as in a religious or political movement, can also lead to crystallisation of thought and an inability to progress.

The ability to let go and to move forward, taking only those things which are still relevant to the present day is one of the greatest healing forces within the universe.

Disease is often seen as a crisis in one's life and yet the word "crisis" comes from the Greek word "*krisis*", a decision. This is a turning point; the decision to be made is to turn from one aspect of polarity which is being expressed in an extreme manner and to face, experience and accept the other.

Sometimes the need for balance and equilibrium is seen on a wider scale and will be reflected in the appearance of "crisis" within the lives of a number of people at the same time.

The method by which the earth deals with such a crisis is seen in terms of natural disasters such as erupting volcanoes, typhoons and earthquakes where excess energy is released in order to redress the balance.

The physical body maintains a harmonic environment (homoeostasis) by detecting imbalances at an early stage and, by fine tuning, correcting them without the problem being brought into conscious awareness.

However, when the influence of the mind overrules these adjustments, then the imbalance can reach crisis point and disease is inevitable in order to recreate harmony.

Once both poles of existence have been accepted then their influence upon our learning becomes negligible. It could be said that through unity their collective note is in harmony with the individual's soul.

For example, in health, we do not have to concern ourselves that the contraction of the muscles of the heart will not be followed by relaxation or that inspiration will not follow expiration.

This state of acceptance can also be called "*habituation*" and allows the brain to release that which is accepted and known and to concentrate only on the more important facets of life.

GROWTH OF CONSCIOUSNESS

The consciousness of the individual develops through constant movement between two poles of existence. These are initially found within each aspect of the personality; the physical, the emotional and the mental.

Through experiencing and observing the different levels of duality and accepting their existence, the individual soon comes to realise that they are not separate entities but a continuum around a common aspect of life.

The separation of the soul from each mode of existence is not achieved without some degree of suffering, pain and grief. For many, these extreme states act as a springboard for action.

A deep depression is known as "the dark night of the soul". Here there is often a state of numbness or the individual exhibits automatic actions. But it is at this time that the light of the soul can be seen. For in a lighted room, the flame of a candle is easily missed. but in a dark room the candle throws out tremendous light.

Extremes are tiring and hopefully through understanding it will become unnecessary to stay in one extreme aspect whilst attempting to avoid the other.

This is particularly appropriate in the case of the emotions where the suppression of one emotion allows it to build inside until its release is explosive and un-contained. Inevitably this then leads to further fear of this emotion and further suppression.

I commonly see this in men who have chosen to suppress their anger in an attempt to appear in control. All that happens is that their rage builds until it explodes into action thus creating further problems.

The psychologist, Jung, called the unexpressed pole of duality the "shadow side" and explained that in continually running from this aspect we are only creating a greater shadow. He advised that we should face it as a friend.

Symbolically there is no shadow when we stand directly under the sun. It is only when we place distance between ourselves and the sun (the soul) that the shadow appears.

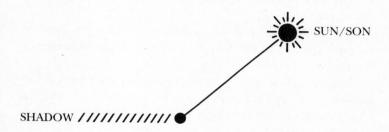

SUN/SON

SHADOW ////////////

Through moving our awareness from the influence of the personality and the outer world to that of the soul, we realise that although we feel pain and sadness, they are passing phases.

The alternative is to remain ever bound to the collective mind of the physical, emotional and mental worlds and never achieve self-consciousness and peace.

An Analogy
A deep-sea diver dons a heavy, old fashioned diving suit and is lowered to the bottom of the sea. His only connection with the surface is through his lifeline attached to his chest.

On the ocean bed he is no longer able to see or hear clearly and his movements are hampered by the weight of the suit.

As his life on the ocean bed continues, his memory of life on land starts to fade and his senses become primed only for life in water.

He wanders around the bottom of the sea bumping into others and asking them if they know the way. Full of their own importance they suggest that he follows them and off they both go, neither clear about directions but neither wanting to acknowledge the fact.

At a certain point, the lifeline becomes taut and our diver is forced to stop and retrace his steps. There he stands looking from left to right, dazed and frightened.

Then with extreme effort he slowly turns and raises his eyes upwards. He can make out a very dim light.

With slow but steady movements he gradually makes his way to the surface, often falling back, but now aware of a force on the other end of the line which is slowly pulling him towards the surface.

He no longer needs the directions of others for he now has his own light to follow, the light of the soul and ultimately of the Divine Source of all Light.

The soul is there to show us the way and to offer support but cannot force us to follow the light. It is within our freewill to identify with the different aspects of the personality or to seek a more fulfilling, though not always easy, path.

THE PATH

The Physical World

An individual identifies with the material or physical world. He is his richness and his poverty; his sickness and his health; his darkness and his lightness.

And yet within these experiences he becomes aware that he is neither and he is both.

For example:

A rich man perceives himself as never having enough and therefore feels poor.

A pauper sees himself as rich if he finds a small scrap of bread.

Ultimately it depends on the level of perception.

As with the concept of yin and yang, words such as richness and poorness are only relative expressions of a situation rather than absolutes.

They are ever changing according to the position of the observer and the further from the site of action, the easier it is to see that these two extremes are two sides of the same coin or more appropriately different positions on a circle.

An Analogy

Two little boys are standing in the playground.

"I've seen an elephant" says the first. "It has large ears and a long trunk which can swing down and pick you up from the ground".

"That's not an elephant" says the second little boy.

"I saw one last month and it had large thick legs and a tail which when it was swung could knock you off your feet".

"You are wrong" shouts the first little boy. "You don't know what you are talking about".

"And you wouldn't know an elephant if it walked over you" retorts the second.

At that moment an older and wiser boy comes towards the two quarrelling children.

"I have sat on top of an elephant.

At the front is a long trunk and large ears.

At the back is a long tail and thick legs.

You are therefore both correct; the back and the front make up the whole animal which is most clearly seen from a high vantage point".

In spiritual man this vantage point is the soul.

Through man's ability to view life objectively rather than identifying with matter itself there is a natural expansion of consciousness.

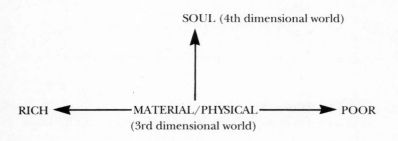

SOUL (4th dimensional world)

RICH ◄──────── MATERIAL/PHYSICAL ────────► POOR
(3rd dimensional world)

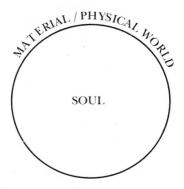

The awareness of unity through diversity parallels the principle of the creation of the soul through the union between spirit and matter.

Here the **Universal Law of Correspondence** is seen to be enacted for this states that all that happens within the spiritual realms will also occur upon the earth plane.

"As above, so below".

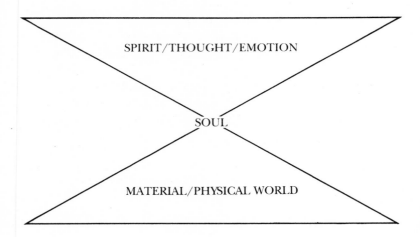

The Emotional World
As man moves along his path his identification shifts from the

material world to the emotional world. He becomes his emotions. (It is never quite as clear cut.)

He is his anger; his depression; his anxiety; his happiness; his fear; his guilt; his joy; his sorrow.

He experiences poles of emotional existence often within the same time period.

For example:

> An angry man at work may never show his
> anger at home because of a fear of
> upsetting others.

> A permanently smiling face hiding a deep
> depression.

> Someone who never complains bearing
> considerable resentment.

Once again it slowly dawns from a vantage point outside the experience that such extremes are unbalanced, tiring and prevent growth. All emotions are only an expression of a thought-form which must in effect lead to action.

We cannot be one or other emotion; they are an expression of the total being and within this there can be no separation.

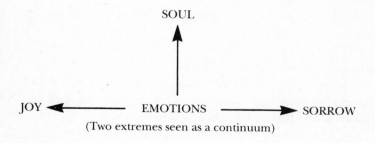

SOUL

JOY ← EMOTIONS → SORROW

(Two extremes seen as a continuum)

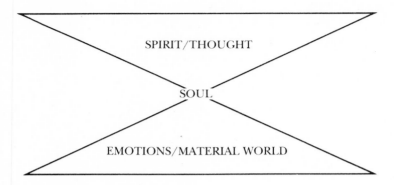

Man is not his emotions.

The World of Thoughts

Man then identifies with his thoughts, his belief systems, the rules and regulations which govern his life.

"I think therefore I am" (Descartes, French philosopher).

Thoughtforms further encompass the illusion of life created by the material and emotional worlds ... we become our thoughts.

In this way our actions become reactions based on belief systems laid down following a previous life situation. In most cases there is a strong emotional attachment which is binding the "actor" to the experience and not allowing him\her to become the observer or "audience".

ie. our emotions create the thoughtform rather than the soul.

For example

When Anne was 6 years old, her father left home to live with another woman. She could not understand why this had happened as she thought that her father loved her.

She came to the conclusion, in a childlike manner, that it must have been something that she did which caused him to leave.

Holding this belief inside, she carried on through life until she started to go out with boys. One relationship after another ended. In most cases the boys said that her love was suffocating and that any suggestions to ease back were met with claims that they did not love her.

She had a desperate need to please her partner for in her mind this meant that he would not desert her. Her need to be loved and her belief that this could only come from another person caused great heartache and distress.

One day whilst talking to a friend she realised that the pattern was repeating itself time and time again. She came to see that her own lack of self-love was attracting towards her those who would confirm her own inner beliefs.

As she learnt to take care of her needs and to understand the pattern of her parents' marriage, she became more self-assured.

Last year she started a new relationship but this time as a much stronger and wiser person.

Thoughtforms and belief systems are laid down in our formative years and are represented by the "shoulds and should nots" and the "do's and do nots" of life.

Throughout life we swing between rebelling and conforming to these rules until we find a balance which represents those beliefs which are still appropriate and valuable to this present age.

Such balance is found by following the Universal Laws of Life and by testing the rules to see whether or not they are still appropriate, accepting the consequences of our actions as part of the learning experience.

Only by using the intuition can we truly know which thoughts originate from the soul and which belong to our personality.

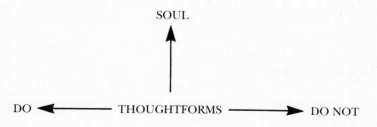

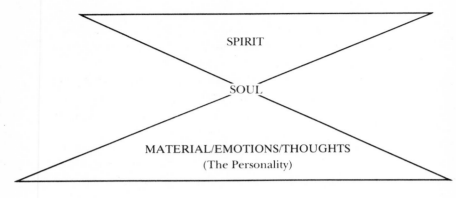

SPIRIT

SOUL

MATERIAL/EMOTIONS/THOUGHTS
(The Personality)

Once man knows himself as a personality and as a soul, the latter becomes the mediator for access to the spiritual planes. The next stage is for the soul to bring its energies down through the personality until the light of the soul shines out of its vehicle.

"First find yourself along the path; then lose yourself and the path is won (one)".

To achieve this, the awareness of the soul is once again tested as it passes down through the mental, emotional and physical planes.

The duality is presented again but this time, with the soul in command, the individual can see those planes for what they are and is therefore less moved by the diversity.

THE UNIVERSAL LAWS

Esoteric teaching states that there are a number of Laws which govern the Universe.

1) **The Law of Correspondence** has already been discussed with the concept that all that occurs on a spiritual plane will also occur on the earth plane.

2) **The Law of Re-Incarnation** states that we do not live only one life but many.

This allows the individual to experience life in all its aspects and hence to enhance the growth of the consciousness.

The concept of re-incarnation was present in the Bible until 553 AD when the Church Council of Constantinople decreed that such a belief should be excluded from religious instruction.

Following this ruling, Western man came to believe that there is only one life with the possibility of an afterlife.

Eastern philosophy, however, maintained the teachings and these thoughts are once again entering the spiritual centres in the West.

The many lives should be seen as expressing the different aspects of the self in an attempt to understand the whole.

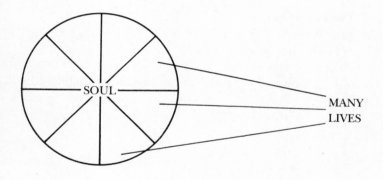

I believe that before entering the earth plane we choose the lessons which we wish to learn in this life.

This means that we choose our parents and our family and subsequent acquaintances and friends.

Our "blood" family are our greatest teachers and despite any anger or hatred towards them, they are difficult to forget. With friends it is far easier to remove yourself from their presence.

Our true spiritual family do not necessarily live under the same roof ... you recognise them on first sight and like what you see. They give guidance and support at times of need and then may pass out of your life.

Whether you believe in one life or many is not entirely relevant. What is relevant is the ability to live in the present time and in the presence of your soul.

There are three other Universal Laws which govern our ability to bring towards us that which is needed for our growth.

3) The Law of Opportunity
This states that the opportunities for learning and growth will always be available as will the tools necessary for the task.

4) The Law of Attraction
This states that we will attract towards us all that we require. It does not however always promise that this is what we want!

5) The Law of Karma
This law states that all we put out must eventually return.

... "As you sow so will you reap".

Just as the tide goes out, it will eventually come in; we breath in and then out; contraction of a spring will be followed by relaxation.

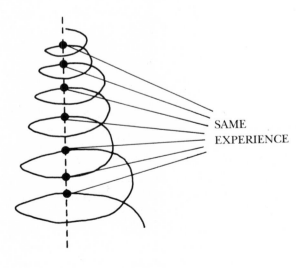

SAME
EXPERIENCE

Karma is not punishment for wrong doing. It is there to help us to understand both poles of existence and to choose to become neither.

If we choose or fail to take advantage of the opportunity before us then in view of the fact that life is a spiral, the same experience will be offered again in a different guise. However there is no guarantee that it will be easier next time!

However, in many cases each time we attempt to "climb over the wall" we lay down another layer of earth which creates a ramp for our final departure from a position of inactivity.

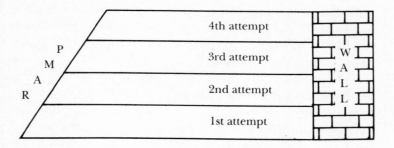

So to recap:
1) In the beginning was the Divine Energy Source.
2) In taking form, this Energy divided into two poles: Spirit and Matter.
3) The union between these two poles created the Soul.
4) The Soul expresses the degree of consciousness released through the union.
5) The purpose of life is to increase the level of consciousness which occurs through the interaction between spirit and matter.
6) The purpose of man is to develop self-consciousness, ie. to see himself as separate from his personality and then to lose this separation as the energies of the soul and personality merge to form spiritual man.
7) This increase in consciousness is achieved by experiencing and accepting various aspects of duality and recognising first their differences and then their sameness.

8) In this way man can start to see himself as both spirit and matter and then to see that they are from the same source.

9) One of man's greatest areas of friction to these ideas is in the field of the emotions or the desires.

10) Disease within the physical body is often the means by which the balance is redressed.

Exercise 1

1) Choose 6 things which you like about yourself, eg. your nose, your laugh, your caring nature, your ability to listen, your sensitivity and your ability to mix well with other people.

2) Choose 6 things which you do not like about yourself (much easier!). eg your hips, your intolerance, your irritability, your moodiness and desire to be left alone, your love of chocolate and your bad skin.

3) Now affirm to yourself in a mirror or to another person your good points; "I like my ..." or "I like the fact that I am ..."

4) Now affirm to yourself or another that the negative points are part of your total being; "I accept my ..." and if possible "I love my ..."

5) Now look at the two lists and see if there are areas of contradiction:

"I am caring ... but intolerant".

"I like mixing with people ... but I want to be left alone".

"I love chocolate ... but I hate my bad skin".

These examples show areas of conflict around a common theme. To hate the negative points is missing the point. Their existence represents an area of imbalance.

In the above example, an over-caring nature can mean inadequate time spent in receiving and too much time spent in giving leading to an expression of the imbalance through irritability, comfort feeding and moodiness.

The clue is to detect the common theme.

In this case, poor love for self, except through the identity of the listener and the carer, leads to disharmony.

By finding time for self and becoming aware of the areas where there is neglect such as with the diet ... the so called "negative" aspects dissolve whilst those that are "positive" are harmonised.

Exercise 2

1) Choose 2 people with whom you feel some disharmony.
2) List those things which annoy, irritate or create fear.
3) According to the Law of Attraction, you have attracted these people towards you for your own learning. They are reflecting some aspect of yourself which is still in the shadows.

This concept is often difficult to accept but remember not to look at the deed but rather concentrate on the underlying aspect which is out of balance.

For example:

Your husband refuses to push himself forward at work always allowing others to walk over him. You see him as weak and become frustrated with never having enough money and never being able to go away on a decent holiday.

However, when it is suggested that you perhaps would like to find work, you find one excuse after another. Both of you have a feeling that "you are not good enough" and probably believe that you will fail in any attempt which is made.

Both lacked encouragement from parents and had been told "You'll never make anything of your life".

By seeing yourself in your husband you start to see that your frustration is directed inwardly. It can only be relieved if you banish all excuses and take on some creative activity which is in your reach of success.

In this way your confidence is enhanced and you give your husband a break from your nagging so that he may proceed with his own growth.

Chapter 2

The Subtle Energy Bodies

Man is more than just his physical body.

He has a soul and the soul is the product of the interaction between spirit and matter. These in turn are a product of the Divine Energy Source.

He also has a personality which involves the logical mind, the emotions and the physical body.

These various parts of man are described in esoteric terms as "bodies" and when the physical body is excluded, they are called "subtle bodies" because the latter cannot be seen with the physical eye.

Therefore man consists of not just one body but seven.

An Analogy

When white light passes through a prism, the light is split into the seven distinct colours of the rainbow.

When these colours are once again passed through a prism, the seven become one; the white light:

WHITE LIGHT

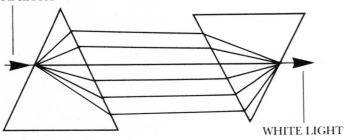

WHITE LIGHT

The "bodies" are interconnecting fields of energy each vibrating at different rates and are named from the highest rate down, as:

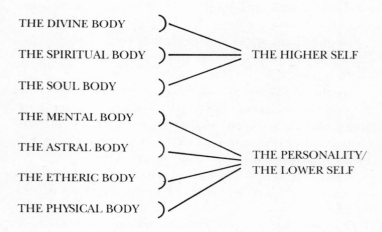

THE DIVINE BODY

THE SPIRITUAL BODY ——————— THE HIGHER SELF

THE SOUL BODY

THE MENTAL BODY

THE ASTRAL BODY ——————— THE PERSONALITY/
                                                  THE LOWER SELF
THE ETHERIC BODY

THE PHYSICAL BODY

The bodies are not found in layers but intermingle. Together they form the "aura" as seen by a clairvoyant.

It is often difficult to conceive that we are more than flesh and blood when brought up in a world in which seeing is believing.

The following analogy may help to elucidate the matter:

An Analogy
If I gave you a piece of ice and asked you to put your hand through it, you may say that this is impossible.

Applying gentle heat leads to the melting of the ice and the production of water. Now your hand can pass freely through the icy water.

If I then said that I can make the water disappear, you may once again question the validity of my statement. However, with further heat the water turns to steam and then disappears into the air.

By increasing the vibration of the molecules, seeing is not always believing.

THE ENERGY BODIES OF MAN

The energy of the higher bodies, the Divine, the spiritual and soul bodies are derived from a small part of the energy which constitutes the Divine Energy Source, the spirit and the soul, respectively.

Few individuals are in touch with the energy of their spiritual and Divine bodies. Such people are usually found among the Holy men of the ancient cultures.

Together the Divine, the spiritual and the higher aspects of the soul body constitute the "**higher Self**". It expresses itself though the "**higher mind**" and is seen to be above daily concerns. It endows the individual with unconditional loving and a non-judgemental overview of life on all levels.

By reaching into the higher mind, it is far easier to see things more objectively and therefore to be able to place them in perspective.

The "**lower self**", the personality or "**the ego**" expresses itself through the "**lower mind**" and consists of the astral, mental, etheric and physical bodies.

The lower aspects of the soul body are the mediators between the higher self and the lower self.

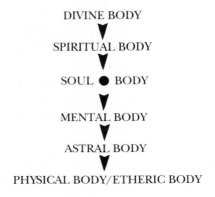

DIVINE BODY
▼
SPIRITUAL BODY
▼
SOUL ● BODY
▼
MENTAL BODY
▼
ASTRAL BODY
▼
PHYSICAL BODY/ETHERIC BODY

In man, the soul chooses the personality which it believes will enable it to take full advantage of the learning situations which are presented in each life.

The various bodies are then brought together by the cohesive force of the soul which is an expression of the power of love.

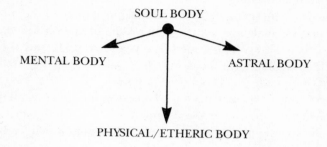

SOUL BODY

MENTAL BODY   ASTRAL BODY

PHYSICAL/ETHERIC BODY

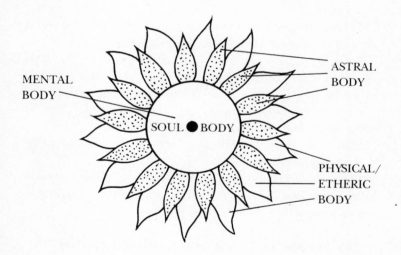

MENTAL BODY

SOUL ● BODY

ASTRAL BODY

PHYSICAL/ ETHERIC BODY

THE LOWER BODIES

These bodies of energy are formed through the original union between spirit and matter. In this way it is seen that they too will encompass their own level of consciousness.

Their development can be seen to parallel the concept of evolution where one stage manifests into the next.

Evolution

In the beginning there was **no-thing**.

There was however the container for all life ... **the ether** (the original female energy).

Through the action of the electromagnetic force of the sun (the original male energy) the **mineral kingdom** was formed.

This kingdom is represented by crystals and rocks and also by the basic chemical elements which are used in the construction of man and all other life systems.

Next came the **plant kingdom**. Plants grow through the interaction between the sun, minerals and the water within the earth.

Following the plants came the **animal kingdom** which feeds upon the plant and mineral kingdoms in order to enhance their species.

Then came **man**; man is an omnivore; his survival is based upon the existence of the other three kingdoms.

To complete this picture of evolution, man should be seen as a small part of the total hierarchy whose combined energies or intelligence manifest as the **Divine Energy Source**.

The energy released from the food of each group is used to enhance the inhabitants of the higher kingdoms.

Man is therefore the collective energy of the mineral, plant and animal kingdoms.

When this is related back to the formation of the personality, it is seen that the "intelligence" of each kingdom is used in the creation of the lower bodies:

a) **The physical body is from the mineral kingdom**
b) **The etheric body is from the plant kingdom**
c) **The astral body is from the animal kingdom**
d) **The mental body is from the human kingdom and is the seat of the will of man's soul**

However, nothing is static in this world and the goal of each kingdom is to attain a higher level of consciousness.

Therefore it is seen that not only are minerals capable of storing and transmitting energy but, through the modern use of crystals in healing as well as in the field of technology, they can also act as transformers of energy which is the function of the etheric body.

The plant kingdom traps and transforms energy from the sun. But in recent years researchers have shown that plants are sensitive to their surroundings and may move away from painful or harmful stimuli.

This sensitivity and the ability to respond to the environment is the function of the astral body.

The animal kingdom is associated with instincts related to survival and procreation but in more highly evolved animals, such as domestic animals, there is an ability to exhibit some degree of individual thought.

In turn man, with his logical mind, which gives him the power of analysis, is aspiring to recognise and accept his soul as a wise and loving being.

THE LEVEL OF INTELLIGENCE AND DISEASE

As man expands his consciousness by experiencing the various "bodies" of his existence, he will identify with the intelligence of each kingdom which will consequently influence his mode of action at that time.

The Mental Body
As yet, imbalances from the mental body are few, since most of the apparent "mental diseases" actually originate from the astral body.

The Astral Body
Whilst man identifies with his emotions he will be linked to the intelligence of the astral or animal body.

This body is associated with survival and hence reproduction. Therefore, in pure animal terms, there is often a tendency towards competitiveness, aggressiveness and defensiveness.

Without the influence of the logical mind or of the intuition, the astral intelligence has a tendency to react without prior thought to the sensory input that is received.

I find that people who are locked into this form of intelligence manifest many diseases whose origin arises from the astral level.

The Etheric Body

Another major seat of disease or disharmony is the etheric body which receives and transforms the collective intelligence of the other bodies and then passes this into the physical body for transmission.

Unfortunately, the intelligence which underlies this body, is not sufficiently sensitive to recognise which electromagnetic energies are harmful to man.

Therefore, over the past few years there is increasing evidence of the damaging effects to health of overhead electricity pylons, underwater streams and electrical equipment in the home.

These effects are seen within the nervous system which is the counterpart of the etheric body.

The Physical Body

Although the physical body often manifests the disharmony or

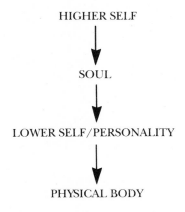

HIGHER SELF

SOUL

LOWER SELF/PERSONALITY

PHYSICAL BODY

disease, it is rarely the origin of the imbalances for it is purely the vehicle for the energies transmitted from the other bodies, manifesting thought into action.

DESCRIPTION OF THE BODIES

The Mental Body

This body is the seat of the will of the soul; the starting point from which the soul can attempt to integrate its intelligence with that of the personality.

It is the seat of logic or analytical thought.

It is the place where the impulses of the higher self, under the guidance of the Universal Laws, pass from the soul and are transformed into thoughtforms and then into action.

Such thoughtforms may occur during sleep, in the form of dreams, during meditation, as a daydream or may slowly develop as an idea which enters the conscious mind as an achievable goal.

To a certain degree, the individual has the opportunity to deny the thoughtform and to bury it in the deep recesses of the sub-conscious mind. However, if this impulse is important to soul growth then it will be offered at different times and in different ways until it is manifested into action.

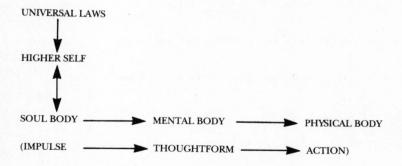

UNIVERSAL LAWS

HIGHER SELF

SOUL BODY ——————▶ MENTAL BODY ——————▶ PHYSICAL BODY

(IMPULSE ——————▶ THOUGHTFORM ——————▶ ACTION)

I know there have been times in my life when I have avoided a particular impulse which has usually involved some degree of change only to find that, slowly but surely, I have been "persuaded" to move by external events.

For example, one morning on going out to the car, I found that one of the tyres had a puncture. Annoyed that this would delay the start of my day I proceeded to change the wheel. At that moment, the telephone rang in the house and, on going to answer, I was invited to a meeting which ultimately led to major changes in my life.

I believe that nothing happens by chance ... if you wish to believe in coincidences ...that's fine ... but you may be missing some golden opportunities!

New ideas need fresh soil. Therefore, before an idea is manifest in the physical world, time may be required to prepare the earth and to remove old roots or weeds which may stifle the growth of the seedling. This is the concept of "Spring-cleaning" when that which is old, and no longer valuable to the present life, is released to make way for the new.

In spiritual man the response to the manifested action is fed back through the mental body where it is given form through the use of memory. It then passes to the soul where wisdom is applied and the results are then compared with the original impulse.

The outcome of the action and the assessment by the soul governs the "character" of the next impulse.

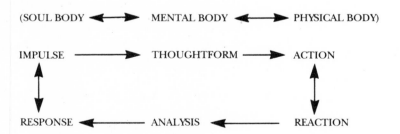

The soul's assessment is based on intuition which is influenced by the power to discriminate. Pure logic on the part of the mental body tends to rely on judgement which is usually biased in favour of the personality.

When man is purely identifying with his mental body, there is little impact from the soul's energy.

Therefore the results from an action are analysed into a "black and white" response and are granted the position of rules. These rules form the basis of "belief systems" which are then the main impulse for future activities.

Rules and laws are not necessarily laid down to make life difficult; they are fact.

For example:
It is fact that if you choose to walk in the middle of a busy motorway there is a good chance that you will get hurt.

It is fact that fire burns.

It is fact that if you do not eat you will eventually die.

Rules are there for our protection. If we go outside the law, then our safety and survival cannot be guaranteed.

The first rules laid down are those provided by parents, guardians and teachers who essentially wish to offer protective guidance within the earthly environment.

Such rules are often accompanied by the words "should and should not" or "must and must not". They teach us about the danger of fires, of roads, of walking too near the edge of a cliff, of talking to strangers, and this advice is good and helps us to feel secure.

Unfortunately, in many cases the rules are flavoured with the biases, the emotions and the experiences of the adviser and therefore the rule does not follow a logical pattern.

For example:
"If you are not quiet, then I will not love you".

"If you do not stop crying, then you will miss supper".

"You should not/must not talk, speak, act, like that".

"Why?"

"Because I say so!"

"Do not let the neighbours know our business".

"Keep it in the family".

"Be a brave little boy".

"Grow up" ...often said to a two year old when the newest baby arrives home.

"Go and play on a motorway!" ...said in apparent jest!

"You should have done better".

"You must try harder".

These are often described as family sayings or mottoes and, as belief systems, may influence the recipient for the rest of their life.

Other sayings, which are meant to be helpful, may be misunderstood by a child whose mind is unable to differentiate one application of the law from another.

For example:

I remember hearing of a child who became hysterical when he was placed in a plastic humidity tent which is the treatment for croup.

When eventually he was taken out of the tent and calmed down he said that his mother had always warned him against placing his head in a plastic bag.

Another child became hysterical when being told that, in order to have his tonsils removed, he would be put to sleep.

It was then revealed that the previous week he had gone with his mother to have his dog "put to sleep" by the vet.

Logical thought develops with age and experience and therefore children often take things at face value until told otherwise.

Seven Year Cycles of Life

The most vulnerable time of an individual's development is the first seven years of life. It is during this time that mental processes are formulated and the basic rules of life are laid down.

Without an adequate spiritual link, many erroneous belief systems become the ground on which the concept of self-consciousness is based.

One of the main reasons why this occurs is that during these formative years, a child is totally dependent on its guardians or parents for food, warmth, clothing and love. He or she cannot go out to earn a living.

Therefore, if a child is told that he will not receive food unless he is quiet, then he will be quiet.

If he is told to be brave and not to cry and then he will be loved, then he will not cry.

Such belief systems are stored in the memory and years later may still influence the actions of the individual.

There will come a time, however, when it is necessary to challenge the wisdom of these beliefs and to see whether they still hold true in the present environment and are in harmony with the individual's own inner truth.

If there is disharmony then conflict develops which in the teenage years is described as the "rebellious stage".

Here the young person is trying to determine what is true for the individual and what belongs to their parents.

They may go overboard with wild hair-styles, outrageous friends and unrecognisable music. This is their attempt to present the other pole of existence to that expressed by their parents.

Between 14 and 21 years they tentatively formulate their own belief systems and apply them in the years between 21 and 28.

By 28 years they re-introduce certain of their parents standards which now appear to have some relevance and combine these with their new belief systems.

However, there are many individuals who pass quietly through the teenage rebellion, only to see it emerge in their 40s and 50s.

Hair-styles change (even though hair may be at a premium), wardrobes are re-equipped and there may be a change in partners or jobs.

In astrological terms such changes follow the seven year cycles of the planet Saturn, which is the planet linked with the power to restrict, but through this to learn. It could be said that at this time we review all those things which are holding us back and choose whether or not we are ready to change and to let go.

Starting Out Afresh

Setting out new parameters from which to work can often appear quite daunting as the "tried and tested" feel familiar and comfortable.

There is often a fear of "going behind the adviser's back" especially if the latter is a parent. There may also be a fear of failure and of trusting one's own new instinct.

The words "I told you so" or "don't say I didn't try to warn you" are not helpful when we are setting out alone.

When the belief system involves repeated messages concerning one's self-worth, it can be very hard to start to develop some degree of self-identity and self-valuation.

The only role left to such an individual is often that of believing that all that happens is their fault and that they will never succeed in anything that they attempt.

As they begin to develop a small degree of self-worth, they may even feel guilty for denying that which they have believed for so long.

They can become both the victim and the victimiser and growth becomes static.

In truth, they are the only person who holds the key to unlock themselves from their gaol ...many can offer support but the "victim" needs to unlock the door to allow friends to enter.

Everything takes time and one of the ways of sabotaging any forward movement is to set the goals too high and therefore fulfil the subconscious belief that nothing is possible.

Whatever the reason, it is often difficult to change the "record" or belief system which is stored in the memory bank and to replace it with a new one.

However, if the time is right, change will occur, in compliance with the Law of Balance and Equilibrium, and we can go willingly or kicking and screaming!

I can think of a number of 50 and 60 year old men and women whose actions are still ruled by the belief systems of their parents.

How they should act; what they should wear; how hard they should work; what they should read; what they should eat.

All sensible and good advice at the time, but which may not be appropriate now.

Whenever I hear the words "Should, ought or must", I know there is a problem.

It begs the question:

… "Who says"?

… "the answer is rarely "I say".

It is far more common to be a throw back to childhood when love, food, warmth and clothing were conditioned by obeying the family rules.

For example:

Maria was a successful 55 year old woman who was a perfectionist. She worked all hours and then wondered why her mind was overactive and prevented sleep.

We talked about relaxation and recreation and she said that this was not part of her schedule as this meant that valuable time was lost.

I asked her about the source of this strong work ethic and she told me that her mother had always told her that she would never be any good at anything.

For the last 50 years she had tried to prove her wrong.

She was not capable of looking at her own achievements and congratulating herself …she still sought approval from her mother.

During times of change it is perfectly valid to go back to old patterns of behaviour for short periods until the new paradigms are well "worn in" and the old belief systems no longer fit the new image.

Deepak Chopra in his book "Quantum Healing" states how difficult it is to change old patterns of a lifetime …not impossible but it requires a "quantum leap" in thought which means letting go and trusting.

Laws and Rules

Laws of the universe and of the land in which we live are there to prevent chaos and to offer security.

Rules and belief systems, however, need to be assessed from time to time to check that they are still in harmony with the wisdom of the higher self.

Such wisdom comes through the development of the intuition and will reflect that which is good not only for the individual but also for humanity as a whole.

Chapter 3

The Subtle Energy Bodies ... continued

THE ASTRAL BODY

This body is linked with the expression of one's impulses or desires in the form of the "emotions".

In spiritual man these desires are derived from the soul and enter the etheric body through the heart chakra. However, if there is no firm connection with the soul, the energy passes down to the solar plexus where it is expressed as the desires of the personality.

The energy of the astral body follows the Law of Attraction which reveals that through our emotions we will attract towards us all that is needed for soul growth.

In this way the emotions produce both the actors and the stage leading to the transformation of the impulse into action.

An analogy
The desire of a plant to spread its pollen leads to the creation of petals of a certain colour and the release of a particular scent into the air.

Insects, attracted by the colour and smell, come to feed upon the nectar.

Whilst resting on the plant the pollen becomes attached to the legs of the insect. In this way the pollen is transferred to another plant where fertilisation takes place.

Thus the survival of the plant is assured and the desire of the plant is fulfilled.

In a similar way, we are the creators of our own world in order to grow and to expand the field of our existence.

All that we sense or experience has been created for a particular purpose in our life whether on a personal level or as a member of the human race or of this planet.

The impulse of our inner world is reflected in the existence of our outer world.

For example:
If I feel happy on waking, I will dress and act in accordance with this inner impulse.

During the day I will find that most people I meet will offer a smile and kind words which will enhance the good feelings about myself.

However, if I feel miserable and feel that the world is against me, I will no doubt meet several people who will reinforce my own feelings of self-doubt.

The Transformation of Thought into Action
Emotions are outgoing; **E-motion** is to set this energy (E), or impulse, into motion.

This is achieved by using the different vibrational energies of the five elements (earth, air, fire, water and ether) to manifest the impulse in the physical world.

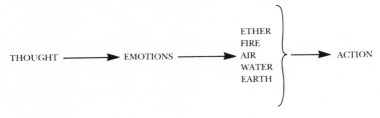

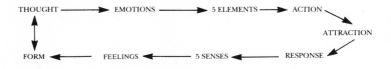

This manifested impulse will then attract a certain response which is recorded by the five senses and linked with memory within the astral body to provide an expression of the message in the form of "feelings".

Feelings are incoming; they are a reflection of the situation.

Through the mental body, the feelings are given form and compared with the original impulse.

The astral body contains therefore both the seat of feelings and of emotions; one could say that which is expressed by the emotions is registered by the feelings.

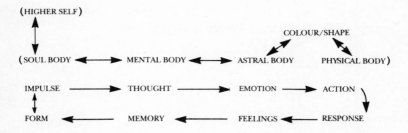

If there is a match between the impulse and the response then harmony is recorded and the consciousness of the soul is expanded.

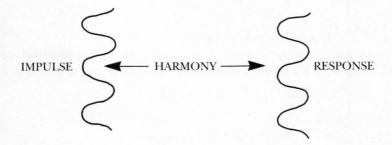

An analogy

An actor plays his part and at the end receives warm applause. He sees the smiling faces and hears the clapping and, on matching these sensory impulses with those stored within the memory bank, he realises that he has performed well.

This means that he has fulfilled the contract which he made when accepting the part and he experiences a feeling of harmony.

However, if the match between expectation and result is poor, ie. the actor does not receive the acclaim or does not feel satisfied with his own performance, then disharmony is registered and the process will be repeated, with alteration in the form of expression, until harmony is achieved.

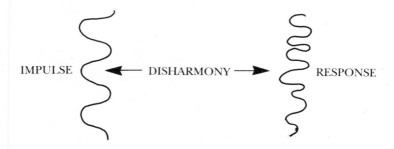

IMPULSE ← DISHARMONY → RESPONSE

The emotions are therefore more than just the verbal expressions of anger, joy and sadness; they also include the manner, the dress and the attitude of the person.

The "Colour" of Emotions

Colour is a powerful form of expression and hence an attracting force. The colours we wear add an extra dimension to the mood of the individual.

For example:

The girl in black may wish to appear mysterious ... or may be in mourning.

The women in red trousers contains much pent-up energy and nobody should stand in her way!

The man with the yellow tie feels vibrant and full of new ideas.
The colours which we choose to wear or with which to surround ourselves in our home reflect those colours which we need for soul growth and which may be absent from our aura.

(It may also reflect the only clean clothes in the wardrobe!)

Apart from colour, the visual senses will also record non-verbal communication which can be a powerful method of expressing a message: A smile, a laugh, the lift of an eyebrow can speak volumes.

The tone of voice, the inflections of speech, the use of gestures, can provide the listener with a wealth of information concerning the state of mind of the speaker.

The Link Between Memory, Senses and Feelings

Stimulation of the senses often leads to recognition of an emotion which is stored within the memory banks.

For example:

The smell of summer flowers may take us back to our childhood which reminds us of happy carefree times.

Conversely, the smell of ether may never fail to elicit the fear of the unknown and of being alone.

Smell is registered in the limbic system of the brain which is the seat of our emotions.

In a similar way, when the other senses such as sound, touch and taste are stimulated, there may be a recollection of a memory which has been well and truly buried.

For example:

White walls may remind a person of the time, aged three, when they were "deserted" by their parents and left in the hands of white, sterile people living in white, sterile wards ... being told that their parents "had only popped out for a few moments".

These children and then adults learn to distrust the words of others, especially those in white coats and aprons.

Such a memory may well influence the individual's ability to enter another hospital or to seek orthodox help, despite serious signs and symptoms.

It should therefore be remembered that memory is only a guide and not law and should be updated with relevant information. As has been stated before, changing the memory of the cells is not easy and requires much courage and perseverance.

The greater the contact with the soul, the easier it is to view things in perspective and to change the "record" which has been playing for years to one which is more in tune with the identity of the inner self.

Emotions are a Necessary Part of Life

Emotions cannot be defined as "good or bad". It should be akin to saying that night is bad or day is good ... which would certainly be untrue for there are many who rely on the night-time for their work.

They are a form of expression which is only relevant to the particular situation in which they are found.

Anger, sadness, resentment, jealousy are all part of human nature. They are part of who we are.

What is more important is that the emotions do not become the ruler of the individual's life, whether they are expressed or suppressed.

Many men and women function from the astral body and never move any higher.

The Basic Problems in this Area Include:
   a) **Over-identification with the emotions.**
   b) **Under-identification with or suppression of the emotions.**
   c) **Identification with the desires of the personality rather than with those of the soul.**

Taking one at a time:

A) Over-identification with the Emotions
Some people are described or describe themselves as being "emotional". This usually signifies that they are easily brought to tears although other emotions may be just as evident such as anger, depression, happiness, jealousy or resentment.

When questioned about their state of health they will reply: "I'm depressed", "I'm happy", "I'm angry", "I'm resentful".

Such a statement, if repeated many times, starts to create an identity rather than just a state of being at that time.

"I'm a depressive"; "I'm an anxious person"; "I'm an angry person".

It would be more accurate to say "At this moment I am manifesting anger, etc.".

Emotions and feelings are there to be registered whether externally or internally expressed and then to be used for the purpose of learning and understanding by the soul.

Once they have been registered they should be released just as clothes are changed to represent a particular situation.

If I feel angry ... I register the anger and then ask myself "My anger represents an energy block which needs to be released. What can **I do** to change the situation"?

This change may be physical or result in an alteration in the way that I view a particular experience.

Such awareness often comes only when we step out of the role of the actor and become the audience, allowing the mind to reach a state of peace from whence the answer will come.

Physically there may not be an easy solution ... grieving is a natural process of "letting go" and needs time ... but there may come a time when grief turns into self-pity. Such a state is damaging to both the "sufferer" and to those around them.

In other cases, it may be necessary to come to terms with the situation and to accept that this is "the way things are" and that such acceptance releases the individual to move forward even though the steps may be faltering at first.

I have seen many cases where over-expression of the emotions hides a fear or resistance to move from a point of the "tried and tested" ... such people are stuck in a rut and this may be seen physically in conditions where there is immobility such as osteoarthritis and some of the neurological diseases.

"I'm too busy being emotional to think about changing"!

Even someone who is permanently "happy" may be avoiding looking too deeply inside for fear of finding their shadow.

This over-identification reveals the two aspects of polarity ...

the excessive outflow of emotions externally reflecting the inner suppression of forward movement along the spiritual path.

Eventually the Law of Balance and Equilibrium will create a situation where change will have to take place.

This may come about through changes in physical health but more commonly through the need to release one's own emotions in order to help others.

Many well-meaning folk have struggled to try to bring a friend, partner, relative or client out of their "emotional" state whether it is anger, depression, jealousy or even inappropriate happiness.

The harder the "rescuer" pulls, the greater the resistance to change. Sometimes the helper becomes the victim, trapped in the web created by the original victim who is now the "victimiser", leading to stagnation of movement for both individuals.

At other times the rescuer marches off in disgust which reveals the underlying motive of the abortive attempt which is to change someone else rather than to look at their own need to change.

We cannot change others or carry them along their path or ours. All we can do is to offer a supportive hand which can be taken within the freewill of the individual.

Many people are very happy being depressed. They thrive on their misery and enjoy regurgitating past hurts and resentments. Just as some people are dependent on cigarettes and alcohol, these people are dependent on their emotions.

By using the principles of duality, those who wish to help such "victims" need to encourage the area of the victim's life which is lacking rather than try to discourage their emotional status without which they would feel totally insecure.

An analogy
If you want to dissuade a toddler from using a dummy, it is best to offer something which is more appealing rather than berate the child for its "childish and shameful" ways!

B) Under-identification with the Emotions

The opposite extreme is the suppressor of emotions.

Such people always start the conversation with: "I think" rather than "I feel".

They answer the questions clearly and precisely although they never mention a feeling. They deal with logic and fact and may even look down on or criticise those who are "over-emotional".

In many cases the emotions have been suppressed due to their reactions to earlier experiences which may have occurred in the first seven years of life, at birth, prenatally (within the womb) or during earlier passages on this earth.

For example:

A child brought up in a household where there is anger and violence may learn to suppress its own anger.

Conversely, a child may grow up amongst a family of "non-expressers" ... not uncaring but not necessarily sharing feelings.

When asked "What makes them angry", the answer to follow is usually "Nothing".

However, if the question is changed to: "Do you ever feel irritated inside?" the answer is usually "Yes".

These suppressors are often the peacemakers; they avoid conflict where possible. They are the "listeners"; everybody tells them their problems ... but they rarely relate their own.

They may feel resentful but rarely complain as there is often now a fear of releasing their own anger in case they cannot control the problem.

In physical terms this anger becomes buried into the liver area and in acupuncture terms creates problems along the liver meridian.

In other cases crying may be suppressed as this was seen as a sign of weakness. The message was to "be strong" in a situation where the child had to learn at an early age to be independent and brave.

Crying, as with anger when used appropriately, is a natural release of energy ... both are part of the grieving process which enable the individual to "let go" of a situation which has been completed and to make room for new experiences.

Restrained tears appear in the physical body as excess fluid as in catarrh which drips down the back of the throat or in swellings of the extremities.

Others fear losing control of the situation through becoming too emotional. The emotions become the shadow which should be denied as long as possible.

But that which is not expressed externally will through the Universal Law of Balance and Equilibrium need to be expressed internally to restore harmony.

Therefore I see cases of skin rashes (unexpressed irritation), asthma (unexpressed speech), diarrhoea (unexpressed fear), fat intolerance (unexpressed anger) and many other conditions. These verify that so much of disease is only reflecting an underlying obstruction to the normal flow of life.

The soul will always attempt to find a method of relieving the system of excess energy either through the physical body or through external circumstances.

For example:
You hate your job. It is boring and this leads to frustration. You become irritated by those around you but do not have the courage to look for a new job.

Suddenly you are made redundant. You are angry with the company who employed you and then become depressed as the days at home drag into weeks.

In desperation you start to sort out your cupboards and find some art work which you had enjoyed in the past but because of pressure of work was laid aside.

Soon you realise that this is more than a hobby and decide to set up your own business selling your own creations.

The energy of the anger has now been turned into something creative and can now be used for soul growth.

Once there is awareness of the block in energy then this can be gently but consciously released without requiring physical illness, external changes or a cathartic experience.

Static energy leads to disease.

Awareness leads to freedom.

Shock

In some cases the strength of feeling which is received in response to the action is so great that the individual is overwhelmed by the experience.

In physical terms such shock leads to a state of fainting or unconsciousness which disconnects the conscious mind from the sensation of pain.

As a medical doctor I can achieve the same result, ie. disconnection using anaesthesia and if I require the patient to remain conscious then I will give only a local anaesthetic. This will result in loss of feeling or numbness and loss of movement or rigidity. However, it is now well documented that although the pain is not felt consciously it is recorded subconsciously.

Such "pain" whether emotional or physical can be carried throughout life and even brought forward from another lifetime.

I believe that the result of these suppressed emotions is seen in the form of physical ailments where there is unexplained pain, numbness, rigidity or loss of movement.

Such patients may require the help of well-trained psychotherapists to unlock the buried emotion and bring the feelings from the astral body, through the mental body and to resolution on a soul level.

Once on the soul level, the individual can see the "shocking experience" for what it was ... a learning process, however painful, along the way to soul expansion and can release the energy which has been blocked for so long.

The Inappropriate Expresser

I remember asking one of my patients who complained of pains in the region of the stomach.

"Do you express anger"?

"Yes, all the time; I'm terrible at work and my family have learnt to duck as the plates fly across the room"!

"What about your mother, do you show her anger"?

"Oh no, it would only upset her. And yet it is she that causes me to feel angry. So instead I take it out on everybody else".

It is probably true that her mother would not understand

the sudden onslaught of anger directed towards her, but the message behind this situation is that it is the daughter who has to change, not the mother.

The daughter described the mother as "pernickety" for whom you could do nothing right. And yet the daughter was still going to visit her mother with the subconscious hope that someday she would receive approval and hence love from her mother.

"She makes me so angry".

Or more appropriately:

"I feel angry at myself for allowing her to rule my life".

Anger is the fire of the emotions; it is the power which will help us move forward. Anger says "You must do something about this situation".

In this particular case the daughter saw that her need for approval from her mother was outdated and that she was now old enough to praise herself.

With this insight, the attitude of the daughter towards her mother changed. She saw her mother as a woman who had not reached fulfilment in her own life and therefore found it difficult to give praise to others.

As the daughter's feelings of self-worth grew, her stomach pains subsided and she was able to give praise to her mother which eased the situation between them.

Other examples of inappropriate expression are seen when a husband shouts at his wife when she is lying ill in bed.

In this case it is not uncommon to find that the husband does not feel angry but rather fearful. He relies on his wife to be strong and cannot bear the thought that he may have to cope alone.

I find it sad that even in this day and age we need to hide our true feelings rather than show our fears and anxieties.

One other group of individuals to be mentioned are those brought up in an insecure or disfunctional household where there are unpredictable mood changes on the part of the parents or guardians which may result from some form of addiction or chronic mental or physical illness.

These children learn to become chameleons changing their

face, clothes and emotions to suit the moods of others. In this way they become depersonalised and often have to assume an adult perspective on life in order to survive and even to take on the role of "parenting" the unpredictable parent.

As they grow they lose themselves further and become total reactors to the outside world. This leads to severe insecurity and feelings of low self-worth. They are wonderful at mimicry and may even take up acting as a career. They become inappropriate expressers as their gift of reading the other person and reacting accordingly may become blurred by the outpouring of their own suppressed emotions.

All members of this group, unlike those who over-identify with their emotions, need to be encouraged to express their emotions whether verbally, physically, through writing, art or other means of creativity.

But it should be made quite clear that such expression must start with the words "I feel ..." and not "You make me ...". Nobody makes us do anything. In the end whether consciously or subconsciously the decision is ours.

The main aim for this group is to learn that emotions can and should be expressed freely and appropriately and then released. Any reaction from those nearby is the property of the reactor and not of the expresser.

If the expresser chooses to take notice of the reaction then that is their choice. So many children learn to suppress their emotions when their expression leads to a flurry of negative reactions.

For example:
"Don't cry ... it gives Mummy a headache".
"Don't cry/be angry ... it upsets me".
"Why do you always have to make Daddy angry with you".
"Please make Mummy happy and be quiet".
"You don't care that your behaviour upsets me".

This is emotional blackmail and can rule someone's life for a long time. For many their desire to please and to be liked over-rules all rational thought. Such reactions threaten the peace and tranquillity of the external world and this is worth maintaining despite the inner turmoil. We must all own our emotions and see them as messengers rather than rulers or jailers.

C) Identification with the Desires of the Personality Rather than the Soul

This is the commonest problem.

The first two examples describe the expression of two poles of existence around a common theme; over or under-expression leads to obstruction, often due to fear, in the movement along the path.

The third problem relates to the registration of the feeling by the mental body but failure to pass the message on to the soul for an objective view of the situation.

The result of this "short-circuit" is that new impulses do not come from the soul but rather from the personality whose desires or impulses are based on belief systems which derive their origin from previous life experiences.

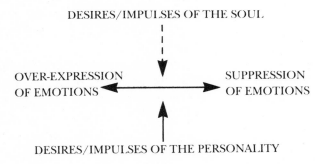

For example:
I believe or think that I am happy. I dress myself in bright clothes and go out into the world feeling happy; I smile and have a jaunty lift to my step. I express happiness.

However, despite my appearance, the first person I smile at has had a bad night and looks and feels miserable.

Due to a lack of deep feeling of contentment, I immediately

take it personally and, despite the happiness that I experienced when I set out that morning, I now feel miserable.

Next morning I go out feeling miserable; I look miserable. Nine people tell me how wonderful I look. The tenth says ... "You do not look happy".

At last someone is speaking the truth!

"I am miserable" ... and in some ways this then makes me feel happy!

Such concepts concerning our state of being are often deeply sown from an early age. Therefore our reaction to each new situation can already be tainted by memory of previous experiences:

"You'll never make anything of your life".

"Stop reading and do something useful".

"Be quiet" ... which amounts to "Don't exist".

"Don't question".

"So you were second, why weren't you first".

"You are bound to fail, as always".

"Your father and I never wanted any more children".

How difficult it is to overcome such deep opposition in order to begin to believe in oneself. To add to the problems, the Law of Attraction guarantees that we will always attract towards us that which we project.

I feel miserable ... I'll attract misery.

I feel happy ... I'll attract happiness.

In the eyes of the soul there is no failure, there is only movement. But within the personality we are faced with two poles of existence:

Success or failure.

Express your needs or keep quiet.

Joy or sadness.

Be active or be lazy.

If I do not value myself, I will continue to meet people who will remind me that I am "no good".

If I feel insecure, I will continue to meet people who are also insecure and are looking for someone who has even less confidence so that they may feel better.

We truly are the creators of our own illusions.

We are stuck on a merry-go-round of acting on the basis of our reactions.

There is an alternative: to look up towards the place of the soul which is non-judgemental and gives unconditional love.

Here we can say: "I may not be perfect, but I'm alright".

Here we can learn to stand back from situations and to realise that other people also have problems. We can then allow them to express their emotions without becoming personally involved.

Here we can see that it is "fine" to express emotions of sadness and joy, to be busy and to relax, to talk and to be quiet. They all represent different aspects of the complex but beautiful organism called man.

Stepping away from the desires of the personality requires the individual to become aware of their own intuition and to become confident of its ability to guide them to areas where there is scope for the expansion of consciousness.

Learning to rely on one's intuition may take time but in the end its wisdom is seen to be more reliable than listening to the judgement of others.

Constructive criticism will always ring a chord with your own inner truth.

An analogy
I am walking along my life path when I come across a beautiful horse which stands in my way. I mount the horse and slowly it begins to move.

Initially I am thrilled by the feeling of the wind in my hair but as the horse starts to gallop faster I begin to feel unsafe. I try to slow the horse by pulling on the reins; but there is no response and I start to shout for help.

The speed of the horse is now so fast that there is no way of distinguishing individual structures in the surrounding scenery and I become completely disorientated.

At that moment someone shouts "Jump". But the fear which accompanies the thought makes me cling on more tightly.

Eventually I become so dizzy that I can feel my grip on the

reins loosening and I fall unconscious from the horse onto the soft ground.

When I come to, I look and see to my astonishment that my beautiful horse is only part of a merry-go-round.

It was all an illusion. Staying on the horse could only take me round and round in circles. The faster the animal moved, the more fearful I became, dis-orientated and out of control.

Leaving the horse, however frightening at the time, led to the re-instatement of control and the freedom to move forward again.

Dis-orientation literally means to be "away from the East". In Native American teachings, the East is said to be the site of enlightenment. Re-orientation leads to re-alignment with our own source of inspiration which is the soul.

Sometimes the only way of moving from a static position to one of freedom and movement is through a thorough shake-up of the original pattern allowing a new design to form under the guidance of the energy of inspiration.

Nothing is ever wasted or lost but sometimes it helps to look at things from a different angle.

We are not our emotions, just as we are not our material possessions or our belief systems. We use our emotions to express the energy of the soul and through this we grow.

THE ETHERIC BODY

The main function of the etheric body is to connect the physical body to the incoming energies of the astral body, the mental body and the energies of the higher self.

Such sources are sometimes termed "the life force" as they animate all life whether human, plant-like or planetary.

The vitalisation of the physical body by the etheric body occurs mainly through its counterpart, the nervous system and in particular through the autonomic nervous system.

The etheric body is described as consisting of a complex network of transmission lines or "nadis" which run all over the physical body in a similar way to the nerve fibres, arteries or veins. Every cell is touched and vitalised by this energy force.

In this way, the etheric body also acts as the blueprint for the construction of the physical body; the force of energy emitted and its rate of vibration determining the cellular formation required in order to create organs and systems.

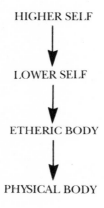

HIGHER SELF

LOWER SELF

ETHERIC BODY

PHYSICAL BODY

An analogy
If I turned a light on outside in the dark, after a while moths would form around the light until all that could be seen was a mass of moth.

Not knowing any better it might be thought that there was no light but just this ball of "moth".

On turning the light off, the moths disperse and nothing remains.

This analogy is symbolic of the effect of the etheric body on the physical body. When the "force" is active, we experience life. When the force is switched off, we experience death.

As has already been stated, the etheric body also links the individual to the electromagnetic force emanating from the etheric body of all lifeforms. In this way a network is created which spans the planet and even the universe.

The etheric body could be said to link all matter whilst the soul body links all spirit.

In recent years, technology has expanded at a tremendous rate leading to the widespread inclusion of electrical and computerised tools within our homes and workplaces. For some people this electromagnetic energy with its positive ions, is creating disharmony within their etheric bodies causing disease especially of the nervous system.

Such sensitivity to electromagnetic fields will depend on the state of the other bodies at the time, but I believe that more care needs to be taken to diffuse the energy of these positive ions in order to reduce the increasing number of diseases now affecting the nervous system.

THE PHYSICAL BODY

The splitting of the atom revealed that behind an apparently solid structure was a dynamic interplay of electric particles all expressing different aspects of the energy field.

With this knowledge, the physical body can no longer be viewed as a solid, static form but should be seen as a complex, synchronised mass of moving energy particles, each giving shape and form to the composition of the body, as expressed by the presence of cells and organs.

In terms of spiritual man, the physical body is a product of, and a vehicle for, the combined energy of the other bodies.

It possesses an excellent range of talents such as flexibility, agility, creativity, regeneration, transformation, extreme sensitivity and a very efficient communication system.

It relies on optimal nourishment not only from the food that is eaten and from the air which is breathed but also on the "intelligent" input from the lower and higher minds.

The appearance of disease within the physical body usually signifies disharmony at a deeper level. Ideally it is preferable to redress the balance at the deepest level possible and hence to eradicate the disease in the physical body. Sometimes, however, the physical changes are irreversible and adjustments need to be made in the deeper levels to accommodate the change.

An analogy

The function of a car is not dependent on the outer form but on the inner workings of the engine and on the activities of the person in the driving seat.

If a wire becomes loose and one of the headlamps fails, then a wise owner will seek the help of an expert who will recognise the fault and reconnect the wire.

However, if advice is not sought or not available then the driver will be unable to drive safely in the dark and this will handicap his performance.

Failure to take note of the initial warning signs may lead to the need for more serious signs to manifest in order to attract attention.

The physical body emits an electromagnetic force which can be measured and used as a guide to assess the functioning capacity of the body. This force is seen in **Kirlian photography** which has been used to outline areas of disharmony within the body. Such photography also recognises the subtle interplay of energies between two individuals who are in close physical contact. This is particularly relevant in the healing arts where the therapist's own energies will inevitably influence the well-being of their client.

Much work is now being carried out to enable practitioners to be able to record the energies emanating from the other bodies.

The physical body is the sacred temple of the soul; without it, our journey on this earth is finished. It should therefore be treated with the respect that any sacred object deserves. It is said that the heart has the capability to survive for 400 years; man can destroy it in 40.

It saddens me that the physical body is used to carry not only all the good things in life but also all our hatred, bitterness, resentment and hurts. These forms of pollution destroy our temple far sooner than any external pollution.

Loving this vehicle is the first stage towards total love and hence wholeness.

THE CAUSAL BODY

Prior to death the impulses of the higher and lower minds are withdrawn causing the disintegration of the etheric body which leads to the inability of the physical body to survive.

The positive aspects of the astral and mental bodies which have been developed in this lifetime form the causal body. Those more negative aspects of our life are transformed into a positive energy to be used at a later date.

The building of the causal body takes many lifetimes and eventually will form the temple of the soul. This permanent vessel acts as the spiritual counterpart to the personality, carrying the soul between the various lifetimes on earth.

THE AURA

Despite the fact that the bodies have been described individually, it should be remembered that they are integrated and that their energies intermingle.

This combined energy is termed the "aura".

To a clairvoyant, the aura is seen as a cloak of moving colours surrounding the individual. The colours will exhibit a variety of shades and will vary in their degree of expansion from the physical form.

The greater the harmony between the bodies, the larger the aura. Prior to death, the aura reduces in size as the life force leaves the physical body.

We are all, to varying degrees, sub-consciously aware of the auras emanating from other people. Where we chose to sit or stand may be due to the sense that a particular person has a "brighter" aura while that of another is "darker" and less welcoming.

In view of the fact that the energy of a healer's aura will influence their healing abilities it is vitally important that anyone in the caring professions works at expanding their own consciousness before attempting to help others.

The Four Functions and the Bodies

The psychologist Carl Jung proposed four psychological functions which represented essential mental attitude ... sensing or perception, feeling, thinking and intuition.

These can be linked with the four elements: earth, water, air and fire respectively and with the four bodies as shown below:

> **SENSING eg. touch, taste, vision etc. ...**
> **PHYSICAL/ETHERIC BODY**
> "I sense ..."
> **FEELING eg. anger, joy, sadness etc. ...**
> **ASTRAL BODY**
> "I feel ..."
> **THINKING eg. analysis, logic ...**
> **MENTAL BODY**
> "I think ..."
> **INTUITION eg. unconditional knowing ...**
> **SOUL BODY**
> "I know ..."

Most people express themselves through one or two characteristic mental attitudes eg. feeling/sensing or intuition/thinking.

We should function within all four attitudes since the suppression of any one function may lead to its manifestation as disease in the physical body.

Exercises:

1) List 3 or 4 family mottoes which you can remember from your childhood;

For example:
> "Don't let the neighbours know".
> "The Devil makes work for idle hands".
> "Don't speak until you are spoken to".
> "Always wear clean underwear just in
>   case you have an accident"!

a) Are these still relevant in your life?

b) Have you passed these messages on to your children?

c) Are any of these no longer relevant?

We receive much sensible advice from our guardians but sometimes that which was relevant as a child is no longer needed. Fear is often the stumbling block. Decide to have the courage to move beyond the out-of-date belief system.

Many times we reject the advice given in childhood only to find ourselves repeating the same statements to our children.

Check to see whether your advice is warranted.

2) Listen to your own conversation:

How often are the words: "should, must, ought to, have to" ... used?

Ask yourself who is giving you the directions? Your Higher Self or the Personality which may still be ruled by the past?

3) Look at the colours which surround you in your home and in the clothes that you wear.

What are they saying to those whom you meet?

Are you happy with this statement?

If not, maybe this is a time for change. Nothing rash, but moving in another direction.

4) Listen again to your conversation for the following phrases: "I feel", "I think", "I sense" and "I know".

Which two do you tend to use when starting a conversation?

For example:

"I think" and "I sense":

As explained in the text, suppression of the other functions can lead to energy blocks which may manifest as physical disease.

Choose to express these latent functions by starting your sentences with "I feel" and "I know".

It is amazing to see the transformation in the content of a conversation just by altering the first few words.

Chapter 4

The Chakras

Within each of the six subtle bodies are found seven main centres of energy or "**chakras**" which are closely aligned in anatomic terms to the path of the older brain and the spinal cord.

The energy within the chakras moves in a spiral fashion much like that of a firework, the Catherine wheel.

The names of the major chakras and their positions are as follows:

CHAKRA	:	POSITION
The CROWN	:	TOP of the HEAD
The BROW (Third Eye)	:	FOREHEAD
The THROAT	:	THROAT
The HEART	:	CENTRAL CHEST
The SOLAR PLEXUS	:	EPIGASTRIUM
The SACRAL	:	LOWER ABDOMEN
The BASE	:	COCCYX and SACRUM

There are many other more minor centres located, for example, behind the knees, in the hands and feet and around the ear lobes. These provide further sites through which a therapist can connect into the chakra system.

The position of the eighth chakra varies according to the text which is read. Some say that it is the energy centre located above the head which represents the link with the higher self and is often called the "starchild".

A chakra could also be seen as a multi-petalled flower with the central position being occupied by the energy of the soul

THE CHAKRAS

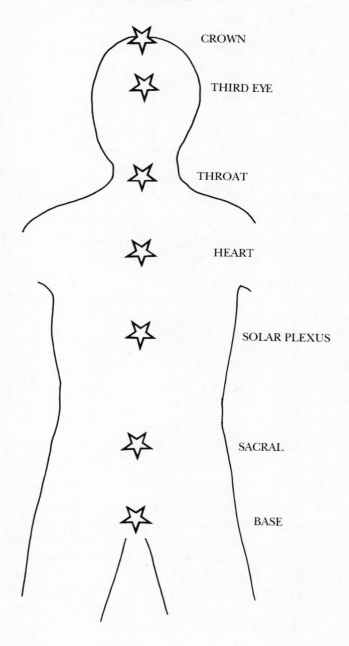

CROWN

THIRD EYE

THROAT

HEART

SOLAR PLEXUS

SACRAL

BASE

containing its links with the Higher Self. From the centre out-
wards, the petals consist of the mental body, the astral body
and the etheric body.

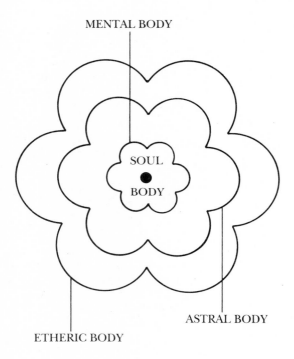

The more open the flower, and hence the chakra, the more
in tune the individual is with the soul energy and the underlying spiritual attribute linked to that centre. The degree to
which each chakra is open, and therefore active, is dependent
upon the level of soul consciousness of the individual and of
mankind as a whole. At present the greatest contribution
of energy entering the chakras is from the astral and etheric
bodies.

Until recently not all the chakras were active, with the majority of mankind working through the energies of the base, the sacral, the solar plexus and the throat centres, ie. those mainly below the diaphragm, while the crown and heart chakras were relatively inactive.

However, the advent of the Aquarian Age, bringing its own energies to our solar system, has led to changes in the consciousness of man through the activation of the heart and crown centres.

This has been expressed physically by an increase in the illnesses relating to the thymus gland which reflects the heart chakra. These include AIDS, allergies, cancer and auto-immune problems.

Schizophrenia, Parkinson's disease, S.A.D. (seasonal affective disorder) and depression are diseases related to the crown chakra and are now medically being allied to the hormones released by the pineal gland. (Illnesses often occur when changes are taking place).

The illnesses have also prompted scientists to take more interest in these glands which until recently were considered to be relatively inert after puberty. Research now shows that several hormones are released from these glands well into adulthood.

The Passage of the Impulse through the Chakra

The energy entering each chakra from the different bodies intermingles until a combined force passes into the etheric body.

This body, consisting of its network of "fluid energies" or nadis, acts as the link between the energy emitted by the chakra and the physical body. Through it the brain and the autonomic nervous system are activated leading to the stimulation of the endocrine glands to produce hormones.

These hormones are then carried around the body, via the blood stream, to particular target sites where the impulse originating from the subtle bodies is manifest into action.

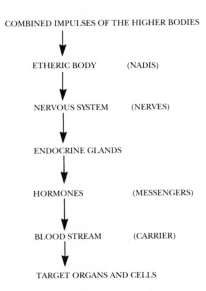

Each chakra is linked with a particular endocrine gland as shown below:

CHAKRA	*GLAND* (RELATED HORMONE)
CROWN	PINEAL (MELATONIN)
THIRD EYE	PITUITARY (STIMULATING HORMONES)
THROAT	THYROID (THYROXINE)
HEART	THYMUS (THYMOSIN)
SOLAR PLEXUS	PANCREAS (INSULIN)
SACRAL	OVARIES/TESTES (SEX HORMONES)
BASE	ADRENALS (CORTISONE/ADRENALINE)

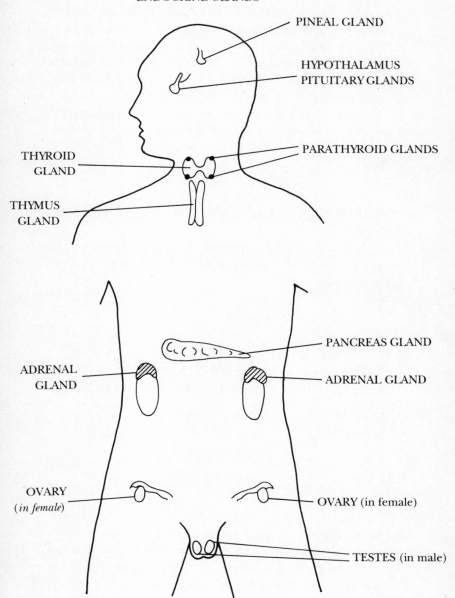

ENDOCRINE GLANDS

PINEAL GLAND

HYPOTHALAMUS
PITUITARY GLANDS

PARATHYROID GLANDS

THYROID
GLAND

THYMUS
GLAND

PANCREAS GLAND

ADRENAL
GLAND

ADRENAL GLAND

OVARY
(*in female*)

OVARY (in female)

TESTES (in male)

The resultant effect of the hormones upon the individual is then relayed back, via the blood stream, to the originating glands. From here the message is passed through the nervous system and etheric body to be compared with the original impulse from the subtle bodies. This comparison then leads to neural and endocrine adjustments so as to bring about harmony between the impulse and the response.

Through this process, the function of the physical body at any one time is dependent upon the activity of the chakras which in turn is dependent upon the energies of the subtle bodies.

SPIRITUAL ATTRIBUTES AND THE CHAKRAS

Each chakra also relates to a specific spiritual attribute which, when combined with the others, symbolises the aspirations of the total human being.

CHAKRA	ATTRIBUTE
CROWN	SELF-KNOWING
THIRD EYE	SELF-RESPONSIBILITY
THROAT	SELF-EXPRESSION
HEART	SELF-LOVE
SOLAR PLEXUS	SELF-WORTH
SACRAL	SELF-RESPECT
BASE	SELF-AWARENESS

The total expression of these seven soul attributes is achieved through the unification and harmonisation of the two poles of existence which surround the attribute. This is brought about by expressing, experiencing, recording, recognising and accepting the two poles of all situations.

The acceptance brings the opposites together in the name of "love" leading to unity.

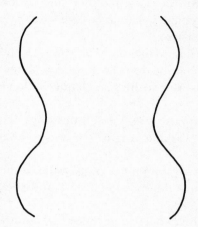

TWO POLES OF EXISTENCE

⟵――――――――――――――――⟶

THE ATTRACTING POWER OF LOVE

UNITY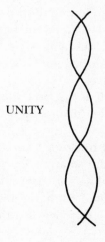

For example:
In the case of the attribute of Self-Worth, I first need to experience times of worthlessness and then times when I feel very sure of myself or could be said to be egotistical or even selfish.

To take the first case:
Someone who has no self-worth or who cannot value themselves often takes on the role of the pleaser, always wanting to help others as this will give them an identity ... they have a need to be needed.

They demand praise even though this is initially in a fairly subtle manner: "Was that alright?" "Is it as you wanted?" "Do you like my ...?"

Unfortunately any amount of praise will not raise the level of self-worth unless the individual starts to believe in themselves.

After a while their constant need for reassurance, and their denial of the support offered, leads to a state of "self-centredness" which was the very thing they believed they could not achieve!

Conversely, the egotist who enjoys being the centre of attention often feels lacking in self-worth unless he commands his space in society. He may need to boost his confidence with a few drinks after which he becomes the life and soul of the party.

This example shows that following the yin/yang principle no state of being is static and each has the potential to transform into the other. Indeed, according to the Law of Balance and Equilibrium, such a transformation must occur to prevent the existence of extreme states.

The ability to value oneself at the level of one's own inner being no longer relies on external identities.

Transformation of the Energies
The base, the sacral and the solar plexus chakras are related to the personality, while the heart, the throat and the crown chakras are related primarily to the soul. The third eye acts as the intermediary between the soul and the personality.

The personality is the vehicle for the soul's journey whilst it lives upon this earth. Therefore development of the lower three chakras is vital to ensure a full expression of the soul's energies.

The Divine Aspects

There are three main aspects required before there can be manifestation of an impulse; the will to act, the ability to create a plan and the ability to attract the tools and materials required.

For example:

I think of making a cake ... **the impulse**

I have the will to proceed ... **the power of will**

I choose or design a recipe ... **the power of creativity**

I collect the ingredients ... **the power of attraction**

I make the cake ... **manifestation of the impulse**

The Will

The base chakra receives the will of the personality.
The crown chakra receives the will of the soul.

The Creativity

The sacral chakra receives and expresses the will of the personality.
The throat chakra receives and expresses the will of the soul.

The Attraction

The solar plexus attracts towards it that which is needed to satisfy the desires of the personality.
The heart attracts towards it that which is needed to satisfy the desires of the soul.
(The power of attraction is the power of love.)
As the soul becomes more deeply incarnate into the physical form, the lower three chakras receive their higher coun-

terparts and the two energies, ie. that of the personality and the soul merge as shown below:

BASE CHAKRA ENERGY MOVES ...
INTO THE CROWN CHAKRA.

Awareness of self as part of life on earth transforms into Awareness or Knowledge of Self as part of the Universal Source of Creation. The will of the personality becomes that of the soul.

SACRAL CHAKRA ENERGY MOVES ...
INTO THE THROAT CHAKRA.

Creativity and its expression, moves from that of the personality to that of the total spiritual being, the inner Self.

SOLAR PLEXUS ENERGY MOVES ...
INTO THE HEART CHAKRA.

Desires of the lower self or personality, which are often conditional, transform into unconditional desires of the higher self.

The **THIRD EYE** acts as the sensory and activating force to guarantee the integration of the energy within all the chakras.

This can also be expressed in terms of two poles of existence becoming one. See diagram (top) opposite.

In cellular terms, this integration is represented by the two strands of DNA (deoxyribonucleic acid) which constitute one chromosome. A chromosome provides the basic blueprint for the structure and function of an individual and mirrors the spiritual design contained within the message of the chakras.

The connection between the strands, which in chakra terms symbolises unity, is seen in the physical body to be represented by the hydrogen atom, which has the atomic weight of one. See diagram (bottom) opposite.

The present increase in the understanding of the genetical causes of disease supports the concept that to correct the imbalances within the chromosomes, by physical means, will lead to perfect health.

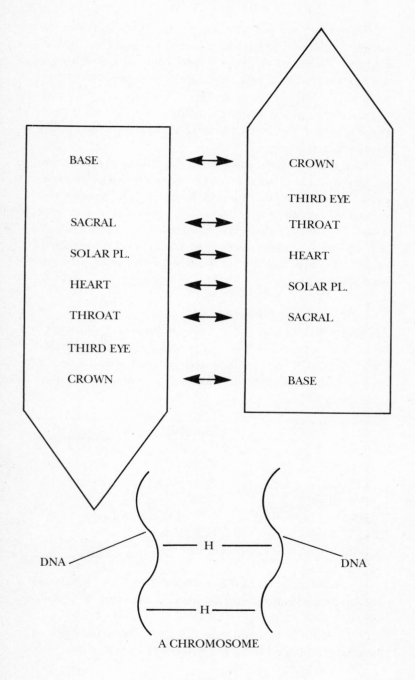

BASE ↔ CROWN

THIRD EYE

SACRAL ↔ THROAT

SOLAR PL. ↔ HEART

HEART ↔ SOLAR PL.

THROAT ↔ SACRAL

THIRD EYE

CROWN ↔ BASE

DNA — H — DNA

— H —

A CHROMOSOME

However, we are still a long way from understanding the deeper mechanism which controls the function of genes. Esoterically, I believe this regulating force comes from the level of the chakras, and that these transmit the energies of the subtle bodies.

True genetical engineering therefore must include aspects of the mind and the spirit and until this happens deeper imbalances will remain.

The transformation phase, when the energy of one chakra merges with that of another, often creates a crisis point in the person's life leading to confusion, frustration and anxiety. This in turn may manifest as emotional or physical disharmony or disease, especially if there is resistance to such a change.

I believe that a more widespread awareness of these natural occurrences may well prevent the crisis point and ease the passage of the energies.

Polarity and the Chakras

Although the chakras contain the potential for unification between masculine and feminine qualities, they can be divided into those which represent the more masculine attributes, eg. outgoing and assertive, and those which represent the feminine attributes, eg. nurturing and receptive.

MASCULINE	*FEMININE*
(CROWN)	CROWN
THROAT	(THROAT)
(HEART)	HEART
SOLAR PLEXUS	(SOLAR PLEXUS)
(SACRAL)	SACRAL
BASE	(BASE)

As you can see, the **Third Eye** is not included in this diagram as it directs the unification of the masculine and feminine energies.

I find that it is commonly the energy in the shadow side of the chakra which is blocked and needs to be released.

I also believe that the points at which the two energies cross will be found to be important areas for treatment.

In the physical body there are often strong links between those areas of the body which relate to the same polarity. Therefore, it is seen that the release of hormones from either the adrenal, the pancreas or the thyroid gland will influence the activity of the other two glands.

Similarly amongst the more receptive chakras. In animal studies on the pineal gland it is known that the hormones released from this gland have a strong influence upon the activity of the sex glands. In man, research is still proceeding to locate neurophysiological links between the pineal and other glands. There is no doubt however that information will be forthcoming, for endocrinology (the study of glands and their hormones) is an ever-expanding science.

Colours of the Chakras

The energy of each chakra vibrates at a different rate to the others. To a clairvoyant this energy is seen in terms of colour and the following guide shows the colours which relate to the particular chakra:

CHAKRA	COLOUR
CROWN	VIOLET
THIRD EYE	INDIGO
THROAT	BLUE
HEART	GREEN/PINK
SOLAR PLEXUS	YELLOW
SACRAL	ORANGE
BASE	RED

While the energy from the Astral and Etheric bodies is a dominant source of the energy entering the chakra, these colours will also be dominant. However, as the consciousness of the individual is expanded, incorporating the energies from the Higher Bodies, I believe that we will see a change in the colours presented at each centre.

Exercise

Find yourself a relaxing position in which to sit or lie, without the risk of falling asleep! Place a notebook and pencil nearby, so that you can record any feelings from the exercise.

Undo tight clothing, perhaps remove shoes and make sure that your neck and back are well supported.

Proceed through a relaxation technique moving from the feet through to the head, relaxing tense and stressed muscles and finishing with relaxing the breathing.

Next, symbolise an energy which represents your Higher Self above your head. Link with this energy and ask that you can be given the wisdom and understanding which will help you to become whole again.

Now, in turn, connect with the energy of each chakra starting with the base. Is there a picture, phrase, colour or feeling which represents this chakra?

When you are ready, make a note of your findings. Having done this, once again link with the Higher Self and then move up to the next chakra.

Continue in this way until you have reached the crown. Then linking with the Higher Self, bring down the energy of this force through the spine, through the feet and deep into the ground. As you do so, feel the ultimate peace and unconditional love which abounds from this source and allow it to enter every cell of your body.

In your own time, bring this energy up from the ground and down from above your head and place the love within your heart. Once again feel the peace and contentment. When you are ready, bring your awareness back to the room by taking a couple of deep breaths and moving your fingers and toes.

If you have a large sheet of paper and some crayons, it is now useful to draw your visualisations from the base to the crown. Using words often limits the concept and you do not receive all the information sent by the Higher Self.

When visualising the chakra, it may be that a different colour appears from the one which normally represents that centre. In this case it is the concept behind the colour which is important, ie. what does the colour mean to you?

You may well be able to analyse your own feelings and pictures but you may find the chapter covering the links between the chakras, the emotions and disease will enhance your understanding.

AFFIRMATIONS AND THE CHAKRAS

The following statements which relate to the individual chakras complete the cycle for spiritual growth:

CROWN: I am fully conscious of, and open to, the will of my higher mind.

THIRD EYE: I take full responsibility for my thoughts, words and actions.

THROAT: I am willing to express my true Self and hence fully participate in my own creation.

HEART: I love myself and others unconditionally, both in the giving and in the receiving.

SOLAR PLEXUS: I am worthy to live my life to the fullest, without fear or guilt, listening only to my own inner voice.

SACRAL: I respect my needs and the needs of others in any relationship and will act accordingly.

BASE: I am fully aware of my position on earth and know that my basic needs will always be met.

When the chakras are in harmony they resonate like a chord of music, the highest chakra of one body linking with the lowest chakra of the next.

Our total structure and function on this earth is dependent on the energy received and sent by the chakras. Linking this energy with psychological and endocrinological functions will, I believe, lead to a whole new branch of medicine, the beginning of which we are starting to see in the science of psychoneuroimmunology.

Chapter 5

The Meaning of Disease

If we accept that everything comes from the One Source, then disease itself must be part of the Greater Plan rather than a mishap which occurs along the way.

So what is the cause or, more appropriately, the purpose of disease? Is it as many believe a sign of failure or weakness? If that is the case, why do we say "only the good die young". Does the fact that you are still here signify success or that there is unfinished business to be carried out upon the earth?

The more I study disease, the more I recognise the complexity of the subject. There is no one cause and each case must be taken on its merits. However, I believe that we are given clues to help us to unravel the mystery. Such clues come in the shape of the presenting signs and symptoms, the area affected, the pathological changes and in understanding the background history of the individual who is manifesting the disease.

Such a background must include cultural, religious and social beliefs whose roots pass deep within the structure of being even though on a conscious level they may have been discarded.

From a psychospiritual point of view, I have formulated the following statements which I believe encapsulate this aspect of the disease state.

1) Disease is just another manifestation of life representing a time for change and opportunities for soul growth. Conscious awareness of the experience can enhance the healing process as long as the consciousness does not remain purely in the head. Every cell of the body needs to become aware of the

changes which are taking place and to release old patterns of behaviour.

(It is not necessary to re-experience these old patterns but only to acknowledge their existence.)

Changes will occur without conscious awareness and may be even more successful as they are then not hampered by the will of the personality!

2) In most cases dis-ease or disharmony appears in the mind before it appears in the body. We can choose to deal with it on the mental level or we may need the physical evidence before we decide to act. Despite warnings, most people do not think that disease will manifest in them.

Physical illness also provides a legitimate reason for one's feelings of disharmony; in the eyes of many, mental distress represents malingering or weakness.

3) If the disharmony is not resolved within the mind, then physical disease appears representing one pole of existence held in an extreme state with the exclusion of the other pole. Such an imbalance can occur on any level and it often represents fear of entering the shadow or suppressed area rather than the desire to stay in the extreme state.

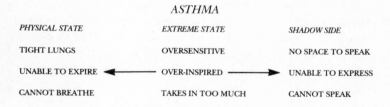

ASTHMA

PHYSICAL STATE	EXTREME STATE	SHADOW SIDE
TIGHT LUNGS	OVERSENSITIVE	NO SPACE TO SPEAK
UNABLE TO EXPIRE ⟵	OVER-INSPIRED ⟶	UNABLE TO EXPRESS
CANNOT BREATHE	TAKES IN TOO MUCH	CANNOT SPEAK

The ultimate goal is to acknowledge and accept all parts of ourselves and with this to regain wholeness or health.

4) The signs and symptoms expressed by the body provide the message that something is amiss and direct the attention of the observer to this area of disharmony.

We can choose to ignore the message by "removing the bulb

from the flashing red light" but in the end the messenger will be heard.

5) The message can be used to treat the physical cause alone or, if there is a deeper psychospiritual understanding, can be deciphered and used to treat the whole person.

6) Disease provides not only a message but also the means by which total harmony can be restored. This may be difficult to comprehend when considering diseases such as AIDS, cancer and multiple sclerosis, all of which are associated with a degree of suffering and a poor prognosis.

However, many people who are manifesting these diseases describe their illness as an experience which changed not only their body but also their view of life, in many cases, for the better.

Until we start to see that health and wholeness must include the mind and the spirit, and that illness and death do not mean failure, we will fail to see the beautiful butterfly emerge from the apparently diseased cocoon.

7) In many cases, the disease is acting as the "spokesperson" for the individual; saying something which otherwise cannot be expressed. When the message is heard, the disease can be released.

Unfortunately, in some cases the message was not clear and the physical changes which have occurred are irreversible thereby providing the individual with a heavier load to carry than is entirely necessary.

These first seven statements could be said to be the "primary gain of illness" which comes from the level of the soul. The next statement relates to the personality and converts the primary gain for the soul into secondary gain for the personality.

8) Here, there is continuation of the illness, despite pain and suffering, in order to satisfy the desires of the personality. The best health care cannot re-establish harmony until the individual can see that, in the end, any gains which are achieved provide little longterm satisfaction for either the soul or the personality.

In many cases, the secondary gain masks much deeper issues

and these may need to be faced before the personality is willing to release its hold on the fate of the individual.

Disease is not a weakness but a way forward.

These statements provide a framework for the study of health and disease. They offer a probable pattern of existence within the range of freewill. They are not given as a judgement or to incite guilt. Such concepts come from the level of the personality and not from that of the soul.

With these thoughts in mind, when I face my patients, I ask myself and also often the patient:

"What is the message and the purpose of this disease?"

It is surprising how often the patient knows the answer but, because they are rarely asked, they have kept this knowledge to themselves.

In truth, the only person who has the answer is the patient and the therapist can only act as a mirror to reflect what is already known but as yet not expressed.

It is not easy to define which particular statement is functioning in each case for, as with most things in life, nothing is clearcut and there are many areas of overlap, especially when group and individual karma are interconnected. However, I hope that the following examples will illustrate certain points in accordance with my thoughts.

The Message of Disease

A) You are late. You run to catch a bus, slip, fall and break your ankle. The physical diagnosis is a broken ankle and the treatment is to place the bones in a plaster cast.

The psychospiritual diagnosis is that you are always trying to fit too many things into too short a space of time and this time you "missed the bus!"

The deeper issue behind this diagnosis is that you only feel worthy when you are busy and hence the permanent running. You feel that you are wasting time if you sit down and that you are neglecting your responsibilities. Your self-worth is related to the degree of visible action.

The broken ankle requires you to rest leaving two options open to you:

a) To use the time berating yourself for being so clumsy, being angry with the medical staff for diagnosing the fracture and to continue to walk on the ankle despite advice to the contrary.

b) To realise that you were careless but that this happened because you are so hard on yourself and never give yourself time to rest.

During the days at home you find that you can organise your day more constructively if you give yourself time to rest.

You learn that self-worth comes with valuing yourself for who you are and not for what you do.

B) Doris was 65 years old when she lost her husband. Despite a large and loving family she was desolate and now had no time for the grandchildren who previously occupied much of her life.

She started to complain of physical symptoms such as shortness of breath and bowel disturbances. But despite rigorous medical tests no physical cause was discovered for her symptoms.

Over Christmas her family became desperate and agreed that their mother should be admitted into a psychiatric unit. By this time she felt her world was black and could think of little else except her own problems.

One day she was coming back from occupational therapy when she saw herself in the mirror. "My goodness" she exclaimed, "What a miserable looking woman!"

From that moment on things changed and she was soon home again with her family.

One month later she had a massive heart attack and died.

I believe that she made peace with herself and was then ready and able to leave this life.

Many strive constantly to change their lives using extreme levels of willpower. However, change often creeps up on us without warning and when we are least expecting it. It can literally occur in seconds but may take a lifetime if we are unwilling to relinquish our hold on old ideas and emotions. The deathbed is the favourite place for making amends and for granting forgiveness, whether for others or for ourselves.

C) Joan came to see me complaining of pain, redness and swelling in the right knee. This was made worse by her daily trips to see her elderly father who lived in a village 10 miles away. Joan did not drive and therefore the journey was particularly arduous consisting of two bus rides and a long walk.

Her father was crippled with arthritis but refused any help from the social services. He relied on his daughter for everything and in the past six months had had several falls which had increased Joan's anxieties concerning his care.

Joan had two children plus a husband and found her days were so busy that there was little time for herself. She admitted that there were moments when she felt that she could not go on and even times when she resented her father for being so demanding. She realised that although her visits were full of good intentions, her resentment undermined her actions.

She resolved to try to persuade her father to accept some outside help and to reduce her visits thereby guaranteeing some respite for her painful knee.

At her next visit her knee was much improved and she told me that circumstances had overtaken her proposed plans; her father had fallen again which had necessitated a short stay in hospital. Following this he had been persuaded by the doctors to accept extra help and Joan now had more time for herself. (I am always amazed by the course of external events which support our decision for change.)

But, despite this good news, Joan looked downhearted. "What do you want to do now?" I asked.

"I have started many things in my life but always fail to finish them", she said. "I fear that I will fail again".

It then became clear that Joan's dedication to her father was not entirely altruistic. It provided a perfect excuse to avoid placing herself in situations where she may fail. She was now having to face her own fears without her father being there to protect her.

We talked about the setting of goals and how important it is to start with targets which are achievable. When I last saw her she had just finished a short course in creative writing and proudly presented her completed article.

When looking at the **message of disease**, redness and pain represent suppressed anger. In Joan's case this was initially towards her father and then towards herself at her own inability to change the pattern which existed.

The site of the redness, ie. the knee, represents humility which for Joan was excessive with a need to "rise from the position of kneeling" and to show more pride in her own self-worth.

The knee also provided an acceptable way out of a difficult situation when words may have given the impression of an uncaring attitude ... **the opportunity for change.**

If the deeper fear of failure had not been revealed then the painful knee could then have been used as an excuse for her inability to develop her own talents in the future ... **the secondary gain.**

Illness commonly masks a fear and may provide the means by which the individual can avoid facing or expressing that fear. Removing the symptoms without dealing with the emotion will inevitably lead to the emergence of further symptoms or lead to the failure of appropriate treatment to act.

In some cases it may be necessary to ask:

"Do you want to get better?" or "What would you do if the illness were no longer present?"

The fact that the patient consults a practitioner is not definite proof of the desire to return to full health. In some cases the ability to outwit another member of the medical profession, or to prove to their family that they really do have a problem, is satisfaction enough and is worth the suffering ... secondary gain.

When I see a patient referred through their relatives or friends and who appears poorly motivated I am not surprised to see that the results of my treatments are minimal.

Other patients whom I find respond poorly to help are those who claim poverty despite appearances and ask for discount on the consultation. It is sad to say that such poor monetary motivation often reflects poor motivation in their healing process.

I have found that in the case of private complementary medicine in the United Kingdom, those who have saved the money to afford the treatment and have been motivated to find a practitioner are often half way to a cure before they enter the consultation room. Motivation is the key to progress and although someone like Joan may be highly motivated in one area of their life, their "busyness" may be hiding a lack of movement in another area.

Here are further examples which I have met in my travels.

a) **A wife pulls a muscle in her back** and can no longer undertake the household chores. Her family rally round, relinquishing their hobbies at this time of family crisis.

As she recovers, they drift back to their other interests and she is alone. The following day she is flat on her back again.

This is a fairly common scenario when attention and love are sought through illness. It is often learnt at an early age when the child may feel neglected due to home circumstances and find that a minor ailment leads to the attention they seek.

With this information now stored sub-consciously, the pattern is repeated into adult life whenever insecurity or lack of love surface.

b) **A successful but stressed businessman is having problems sleeping** due to an overactive mind. He requests sleeping tablets from his doctor but is advised that he would do better to take a holiday and spend less time in the office.

He replies that he has far too many people relying on him and that the only thing that would slow him down would be a broken leg. The following week he falls down …

The internal drivers such as "try harder", "be strong", and "please me" are often so ingrained from childhood that it is difficult to break free and act on the guidance of one's own inner voice.

In this case, the businessman was unable to step off the treadmill voluntarily and circumstances had to take the upper hand. The period spent in bed would provide time to reflect on life and he would probably discover that in his absence others, unfortunately, coped very well!

Nothing happens by chance.

c) **A child with behavioural problems and asthma is brought**

to see the doctor. She is a middle child, between two very verbal siblings. She tends to prefer to go off and play alone.

When the mother is asked about other stresses in the child's life she hints that her own relationship with her husband is not always harmonious and it becomes apparent that the child's bad behaviour is exacerbated at times of the parents' arguments.

Here, the child has become the scapegoat for the family's problems. Such an individual is common in many families ... the butt of the jokes or the receiver of pity.

If the scapegoat decides to change their role, it threatens the basic structure of the family and therefore attempts will be made by the other members of the family to keep that individual in their designated position.

For example:
If the scapegoat is the plump child with nicknames such as "fatty" or "piggy" then everybody knows their place until that individual decides to go on a diet.

Initially there is encouragement until it becomes obvious that the status quo in the family is affected.

From then on everybody tries to persuade this new slim child to eat and tells him that he was much more attractive when he was fat!

If the scapegoat has the strength and the courage to hold on to their own self-worth then remarkable changes will occur within each member of the family until equilibrium is once again restored.

Such cases often benefit from family therapy where each member is given the time and space to express themselves as individuals and not just in the role which they have been given.

They can then start to understand each others' needs and work towards reaching an honest compromise which leads to harmony within the home.

d) **A mother has multiple sclerosis** and is practically bedbound. Apart from symptomatic relief, nothing seems to halt the disease process.

As time passes, it becomes obvious that instead of her children becoming hampered by their mother's disease, they in fact grow and gain from the experience using the knowledge in their own lives in the years that follow.

Positive secondary gain of illness often stretches beyond the patient, affecting family and friends, those in the caring profession and even those who hear the story second-hand.

At the time, it is often difficult to see that any good could come out of illness and suffering, and the initial reaction of the observer is often anger and bitterness.

In the longterm, however, such reactions create their own problems and do very little to alter the initial event. Eventually, conscious acceptance must occur in order to create space for forward movement.

Only in retrospect is it possible to see the wisdom and strength which occurs in those affected by the illness of a friend or relative.

e) **A man who owned a business** always found it difficult to receive help in any venture whether at home or at work. He believed that for a job to be done well, he had to be in total control of the situation. He became irritable and impatient towards those who were slow to understand simple instructions and who made mistakes.

One day at work he collapsed, paralysed down the right side of his body. He had suffered a stroke. His recovery was slow, hampered by his bitterness that his body had failed him.

He had to rely heavily on others for dressing, feeding, walking and even making himself understood through his affected speech.

He became frustrated by his dependence on his friends and family but was amazed by the tolerance shown by others towards him.

I commonly see strokes occurring in those who like to be in control and who tend to be great organisers but poor delegators. To give away such power is very threatening but the body's paralysis necessitates such a move. For this man, it took an illness to gain insight into his own character and, through this, was given the chance to allow others to share in his life in a more positive fashion.

f) **A woman was found to have terminal cancer.** She was hard working and often denied herself luxuries for the sake of her family which she had brought up single-handed following the death of her husband.

Unfortunately, her two sons had fallen out over a business deal and rarely made contact with each other.

When the woman was admitted to hospital the boys purposely avoided each other during visiting time. However, one day they found themselves on either side of their mother's bed and could no longer ignore the issue.

Their mother pleaded with them to talk to each other and because of their love for her they agreed to meet in order to discuss their differences and to see whether they could reach a compromise.

Their mother had never looked so happy.

That night she died peacefully in her sleep.

In this world no action occurs which does not have repercussions on other individuals. All our lives are intertwined and the ability to help others comes from the ability to change ourselves.

Until we are able to see death as a time of moving on into another plane of life, we will still hold the view that it is a time of loss and failure rather than that of growth. This woman had never asked for anything for herself until the evening of her death. Her ability to ask her sons to talk together for her sake was a great step forward and one which allowed her to move to another dimension of life through the door of death and rebirth.

The old adage that "the operation was successful but the patient died", should now be replaced by:

"The operation was successful **and** the patient died".

Psychology and spiritual understanding must, I believe, be part of any undergraduate medical or complementary therapy training for without it our treatments are barely scratching the surface.

The Signs and Symptoms as the Messenger
For a long time the signs and symptoms of disease have been seen as the enemy to be ignored or to be silenced at all costs

instead of appreciating their deeper significance and the message that they bring.

An analogy
If the postman (messenger) brings a tax claim (the message) ignoring him or hoping that he will go away will not solve the problem.

He will eventually make his presence felt using his voice, his hands or even force.

You could shoot the postman but another messenger will be sent. Some people try to bring the postman into their home to make him part of their life ... but ultimately the problem, the tax claim, is still unresolved and unpaid!

The initial problem is to be able to interpret the message which is being expressed by the signs and symptoms of the body. I believe that this can only be achieved through the use of a "wide-angled lens" which encompasses all facets of the individual, including those seen and unseen.

On many occasions the clues are obvious if only we have the eyes to see, the ears to hear and the wisdom to understand.

1) The Spoken Word
I have found that the words which are used by a patient to express their social conditions at that time are often strongly linked with the physical symptoms.

For example:
The woman with a boil within the nasal passages:
 "My sister got up my nose".
The man complaining of an aching neck:
 "My partner is a pain in the neck".
The woman with a bout of shingles:
 "My mother gets on my nerves".
The wife with a burning rash around the neck:
 "I am so frustrated with my husband's actions but cannot tell him".
The mother with severe pain in the lower back:

"I feel that I just cannot take on any more responsibility".
The girl with constant nausea:
"I'm sick to death of my job".
The man with a painful abscess around the anal opening:
"My boss is a pain in the backside!"
In other cases the words which are used to express the symptoms may give guidelines to the underlying cause:

a) **"The rash is so irritating"** from the woman who has become irritated by the fact that nobody carries out her housework exactly to her specifications.

b) **"My hips are stiff so that I find it difficult to move in the morning"** from the man who is now retired and feels that he no longer has an identity in society. Physical immobility often represents mental immobility and the fear of moving forward.

c) **"I am so constipated that I may only go to the toilet once a week!"**; this woman denies any other problems and likes to appear totally in control. She rarely expresses an emotion or a motion!

d) **"My dizziness causes me to be totally unbalanced and I have to lie down"** from a man who lives with an anxious wife, three active teenage children and a neurotic dog.

e) **"I hate myself for the fact that all I seem to want to do is to eat chocolate"** from the girl whose husband has just walked off with her best friend.

In each of the cases cited above it can be seen that the physical body is being used to balance an extreme state which is present on other levels, ie. within the astral, etheric or mental bodies in accordance with the Law of Balance and Equilibrium.

Seen in this way:

a) The woman with the rash is extremely fastidious and likes to see that everything is neat and tidy. The rash represents that part of her which is imperfect and this in her eyes is extremely irritating.

b) This man is feeling insecure and frightened now that he has no specific role in life. Such feelings of being out of control internally have caused him to become immobile externally.

c) This woman has a fear of letting go and of perhaps becoming vulnerable, which causes her to hold on to everything very tightly.

d) This man's external life is so hectic that the dizziness allows him to find peace and quiet within his bed.

e) This girl feel unloved and unlovable and tries to nurture herself with chocolate.

Although all the conditions given above can be relieved through orthodox treatment, I believe that the relief of symptoms would be more permanent if it included guidance in psychospiritual awareness.

Many forms of complementary medicine do in fact look at the whole person in their diagnosis and treatment and can achieve longterm relief of symptoms without the patient becoming consciously aware of the deeper issues.

However, I have found in my own experience that patients not only respond faster to treatment when their condition is discussed with them but also welcome this discussion so that they can take some responsibility for their own healing process.

I have also found that such awareness leads to the patient recognising the warning signs of future disharmony at an earlier stage and that they can then act accordingly to stop the disharmony manifesting as disease.

2) Body Language ... The Visual Message

Throughout the day our eyes register a variety of images, many of which are lost if the image cannot form a useful connection within the brain. Over the years as a doctor, I have learnt to use my eyes, both my physical and my third eye, more and more, not only to study the presenting sign of illness but also to observe the individual sitting before me.

These new images allow me to see the whole person and to treat accordingly.

Many books have been written on the subject of body language and I will only give a few guidelines at present. Much of this information links with my understanding concerning the chakras and will be expanded upon in later chapters.

Examples

a) **A young teacher crosses her arms over her solar plexus (across the waist)** when talking about the stresses involved with her work and the way that she is affected by the plight of some of the children.

The solar plexus is the area through which we receive information concerning our environment especially on an emotional level. Some people who are very sensitive to the world act like sponges, attracting all manner of emotions from their surroundings until they are totally overwhelmed.

Sub-consciously they protect themselves using their arms as a guard against unwanted energies.

b) **A child is deserted by his friends in the playground because he refuses to play their games. He stands with his arms tightly held over his chest and looks sullen.**

The heart within the chest is the area where hurt is registered. To nurture a broken heart or to prevent further damage we once again use the arms as a form of defence.

c) **A nervous interviewee carefully winds her legs around each other in order to feel more secure.**

In this way, the girl protects a part of herself which is often seen to be vulnerable especially among women. A man who sits with his legs wide apart is saying that he is secure in himself and challenges others to come close.

d) **A nervous young boy answers his teacher with his hand partially obscuring his mouth.**

It is almost as if the boy is afraid to let others hear his answer and reflects his lack of confidence concerning his own abilities.

e) **The furrowed brow of a business man warns others to approach only at their peril!**

Non-verbal communication is a very efficient and speedy method of making yourself understood. We are all able to communicate in this manner receiving instruction at a very early age. This is confirmed by watching a baby smile back at its smiling parent and then become solemn when the smile is replaced by a frown.

It is now clear that most babies receive messages from their mother in utero and the essence of this message, at such an important time of development, can shape the life of that individual.

It is no longer appropriate to say:

"Out of sight, out of mind".

f) **The watery eyes of the woman telling you about the death of her husband, shows that the grieving process is incomplete.**

Our actions often belie our words which makes face to face contact invaluable to the practitioner. Such a non-verbal signal needs to be explored, carefully and with the full co-operation of the patient.

g) **The foot of a man jerks as the practitioner asks him to speak about his marriage.**

Such movements are usually involuntary and it appears that the sub-conscious is now joining in the conversation.

h) **A boy clenches his hands together until the knuckles appear white as he talks about his anger towards his father.**

The boy's hands are acting out a subconscious scene where their combined strength would be sufficient to strangle the father. Thankfully his conscious mind prevents such an action but nobody is left in any doubt as to the depth of his feelings.

All these signs give important clues to those who can see and can combine what they see with wisdom. It is not the place of the practitioner to overstep the boundaries set by the patient in his enthusiasm to promote his own ego.

It is easy to offend people by innocently commenting on their words and actions. They may then feel vulnerable and even judged and may refuse to co-operate with further questions. It is also wise to take all the evidence into account before making a decision as to the possible cause of the problem.

Man is a complex animal and over many years learns to apply one layer of behaviour on top of another until his appearance is similar to that of an onion! In view of this, we should all strive to find the inner core of the problem and not be tricked by the outer covering.

The following chapters reveal other ways in which the message can be deciphered, through the pathological signs and through an understanding of the chakras.

Chapter 6

Disease Through the Chakras

Each chakra is related to the adjacent area of the physical body with a few exceptions which will be discussed below.

When disharmony occurs, it usually affects a number of centres but it is common to find that one centre is predominantly involved, with the bulk of the signs and symptoms being found in this area. Following the balancing of this centre, the others may be sent out of balance and require tuning to the new vibration.

In today's world much disease relates to the lower chakras which highlights the problems facing the individual of retaining a true sense of spiritual identity whilst maintaining an acceptable position in society.

As has been stated earlier, many problems of spiritual man are still focused in the astral body and expressed as physical disease. Therefore the chakras are described in terms of their spiritual and emotional qualities and the way in which the latter can be transformed into a new level of awareness.

Chapter 7

The Base Chakra

THE BASE CHAKRA	
Position	: Base of Spine
Spiritual Aspect	: Self-Awareness as a Human Being
Basic Need	: Security, Confidence
Related Emotions	: Fear and Courage
Endocrine Gland	: Adrenal (Cortisone)
Associated Organs	: Kidneys, Bladder, Rectum, Vertebral Column, Hips
Colour	: Red

Anatomy of the Kidneys

The kidneys start life within the pelvis. It is here that the soul lays down the blueprint for the structure and the function of the kidneys during this incarnation, ie. they contain a base chakra energy. Prior to birth they ascend to their normal position in the loins.

The Adrenal Glands

These glands are situated on the superior aspect of the kidneys. Their primary function is to maintain the body through periods of stress by regulating the supply of energy to the essential organs without compromising the overall activities of the body.

Each gland consists of two parts:

a) The **medulla** which is connected to the autonomic nervous system and secretes **adrenaline and nor-adrenaline**.

b) The **cortex** which secretes **cortisol, aldosterone and small amounts of the sex hormones**.

The initial response to stress sees an increase in the secretion of adrenaline into the system which then prepares the body for the **"fight and flight"** response. This is an animal reaction to danger and is a perfect example of duality, providing the individual with the choice to run away or to stand and fight.

The effect of adrenaline is to reduce the activities and the blood supply to the non-essential organs such as the sex organs, the digestive system and the urinary tract, and to divert the energy to the more essential organs such as the heart, lungs, brain and muscles.

Once the danger is over, the body naturally reverts to a position of rest as is seen in a sleeping cat following a particularly hectic chase after birds in the garden. Now, the blood is restored to the non-essential organs and reduced in those which have been previously working overtime.

However, in this day and age, little time is allocated for such luxuries as rest, with the end result that the adrenal gland is under constant stimulation.

This leads to the present increase in muscle fatigue, heart disease, tiredness, peptic ulcers, infertility and digestive disorders.

In an attempt to provide more energy for the flagging system, **cortisol** is released facilitating the breakdown of the energy stores from the muscles and from the liver. However, if the secretion of cortisol continues unabated, signs and symptoms similar to those seen after the long-term ingestion of artificial steroids, start to appear. These include hypertension, diabetes, muscle weakness, thinning of bones and skin and a lowered immune system.

Eventually, the function of the adrenal glands starts to fail and an individual is left with an underactive adrenal system and lowered resistance to stress.

To understand the process which underlies this continual strain upon the body, it is helpful to study the area of soul growth which is influencing the base chakra.

Spirit into Matter

When the total energy of the Soul reaches the base chakra, it could be said that the soul is now fully incarnate into the physical body and that the soul/sole (of the foot) is now touching the earth.

The base chakra is the site where spirit wholly unites with matter and is the place where the **"Will-To-Be"** is formulated, ie. A human Be-ing.

The starting point for the soul's descent into matter is the crown chakra. In anatomical terms, the link between the crown and the base is via the spinal cord which is encased within the vertebral body. The cord, as part of the nervous system, is in direct communication with the etheric body and through this with the other subtle bodies.

It therefore provides the framework upon which the life of man on Earth is constructed. Such a construction is not static for as the soul descends into matter, it alters the vibration of this substance, creating changes in the spinal cord and the connecting nerves, which in turn alter the vibration of the tissues which they supply.

The work of chiropractors and osteopaths aims to realign the bones of the vertebral column and in this way to provide a clear passage for the soul's energy.

Spiritual Aspect ... Self Awareness

When the soul is incarnate into the physical body, there is an awareness of oneself as a child of the union between the Father and the Mother. This leads to a feeling of security, knowing who you are and how you fit into the Greater Plan.

Without such awareness it is easy to feel insecure. To relieve this anxiety, we can gain security by surrounding ourselves with external structures such as homes, families, jobs, etc. This leads to a greater identification with the physical world rather than with that of the spiritual world.

In the base chakra, the issues around security lead to the extreme poles of **superiority and inferiority** which can be expressed as the **fight or flight response**.

Soul growth encourages us to relinquish our attachment to these outer forms and to start to become aware of our own inner strengths. This is achieved by accepting the usefulness of both extremes of existence and combining them to find a less

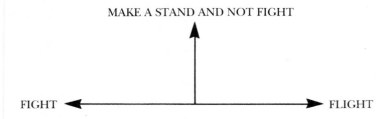

MAKE A STAND AND NOT FIGHT

FIGHT ← → FLIGHT

stressful way of life. This does not include running or fighting. This is known as a passive demonstration of strength and it is seen that animals respect the sanctity of such a move.

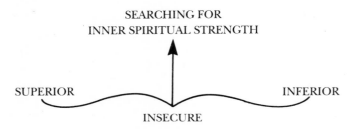

SEARCHING FOR
INNER SPIRITUAL STRENGTH

SUPERIOR   INFERIOR

INSECURE

This statement of oneself requires courage and faith and during its conception may cause many swings towards one or other aspect of the fight and flight response. This is normal and will in time find its own balance if it is not restricted by fear on the part of the individual.

Fight and flight will usually be present at the same time although one will be dominant.

Those who are working to balance the base chakra are often perfectionists, fearing failure and competing to reach a goal which they believe will give them security. Unfortunately, it is not always clear what is meant by perfection and their goals are commonly indefinable, and therefore unobtainable, which leads to further feelings of failure.

They strive to achieve, for this is a measure of their success. To this end, they drive both themselves and others especially at times of added stress. They are critical and intolerant of others who do not work to their specific standards as in some way this reflects their own failure. Unfortunately, such success achieved at the cost of pain to others rarely brings inner peace.

Perfectionists can become irritable and aggressive, appearing insensitive to the needs of those who surround them. When trapped, they may attack or adopt a defensive role, crying or withdrawing from company.

They are often competitive, both in their work and in their leisure pursuits, enjoying sports such as squash, jogging, tennis, swimming, etc. and may become paranoid if they feel that their superior position is threatened by another person.

They have often been brought up in a family where success was valued and love was attached to this success. Here, the mental driving force was "be perfect" and unless this command is released is carried throughout adult life.

There are particular problems where the message received has been one of negativity relating to the fact that the individual "will never be any good" or that he/she "will always fail". This is common where a parent is also insecure and does not wish that the child should overtake them by becoming more successful and fulfilled.

Base chakra people find it difficult to rest for fear that they may miss an opportunity on the ladder to success; they are always busy "doing something". Even when they are sitting they fidget and their mind is overactive. There is never enough time and they are intolerant of queues and waiting. They would rather go without than wait.

They live in the future and the past, missing out on the pleasures of the present. You can recognise them walking along the street; their head is forward already at work planning the day ahead; their legs and bottom are dragging behind in the past, still attached to the happenings of the morning before they left home.

There is only one area in the present, the solar plexus, the seat of the emotions which is busy trying to assimilate the mass of information which it receives.

They have a desperate need to be in control and may be fastidious with their belongings; straightening pictures, indexing records and becoming agitated when someone replaces a book on the shelf in the wrong order.

They work by the rules, placing people and objects in boxes. Here they are safe; they know where they stand and can feel secure. However, if anything or anybody dares to disturb their carefully controlled environment (even if the weather dares to change) then they become irritable and anxious. They do not cope well with change and yet their quest for perfection places them in an ever-changing environment. This leads to a constant need to place a finger on the stress button so that they are ever alert to the dangers of the world.

Despite their perfectionist nature at work, they may live in a slum at home. This reveals the two poles of duality, the latter being expressed to balance the extreme nature of the former. This could be represented by the strict disciplinarian father versus the rebellious son. Neither is totally relaxed and happy in their role as each has to work hard to maintain their position.

The energy which combines both extremes and brings harmony is seen in the little child of about two years old. This child does not live by the rules of man, but of God and remembers how to have fun.

Flight is represented by the need to run away and hide. This may be obvious in someone who has agoraphobia or who maintains a defensive attitude when approached. It is also evident in those who place themselves in a position of authority where they can hide behind a uniform rather than face their own insecurities. As a doctor it can be quite threatening to remove the white coat or to come round in front of the desk so as to become an equal with the patient.

Insecure leaders encourage a following in order to boost their sense of security but cannot allow the follower to become greater in case they take over control. Therefore, they undermine the confidence of those around ensuring a level of dependency and compliance. Such reactions also encompass the energy of the solar plexus where personal ego is stored.

Flight may mean that it is difficult to stay in society and such an individual may become a "drop-out" or a loner. The latter is often critical of others, saying that they prefer to be in their own company rather than that of idiots or bores. By criticising others and hence becoming superior, it is easy to avoid one's own feelings of inferiority.

However, in the end loneliness may be the sole companion. This is not only found in those who live alone but is also seen in those who live in a large family. Many search for the perfect world and reject all that does not live up to their standards leading to tears and bitterness.

It is often said by pessimists that we come into the world alone and die alone. However, I have yet to meet anybody who was not attached to someone when they were born. The umbilical cord provides an important link with our own mother and is symbolic of the link that we all possess, through mankind, with the Earth Mother or Matter itself.

For the soul, a period of solitude can be used to communicate with the personality. Then, the still, small voice may be heard above the crying and the anger. For spiritual man nobody needs to be alone; there are many friends on all levels if we can only learn to let down our own defences and trust. This is easier when we have developed a level of inner strength and security which comes from loving and forgiving ourselves.

Sometimes the insecure pattern becomes dominant and then the inferiority complex emerges. Such people believe that they can never succeed and will always fail. They feel afraid to bring their soul energy down to earth, living partly outside their body in the world of fantasy and dreams and partly on the earth.

The lack of soul pressure leads to hypotension (low blood pressure), dizziness and cold hands and feet.

The phrase "When in doubt, move out" is very apt in these circumstances.

They, too, have problems of living in the present, overcome by the anxieties from the past and by the imagined demands of the future. For them, the fear of living is far greater than the fear of death.

Whether the insecurity is consciously revealed or not, when there is poor control on matter by spirit, diseases emerge which relate to undisciplined energy in the base chakra. These include panic attacks with palpitations, hyperventilation, frequency of micturition (passing water), regular trips to the toilet to open the bowels and muscle spasms. The physical body is out of control.

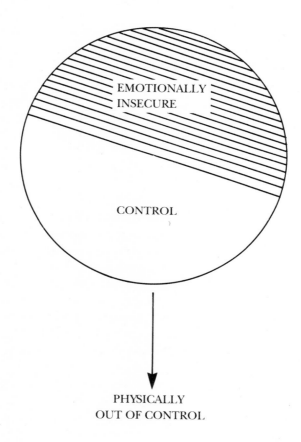

EMOTIONALLY
INSECURE

CONTROL

PHYSICALLY
OUT OF CONTROL

These are all signs of an overactive adrenal gland which is starting to fail. In those who like to remain in control, I commonly hear that symptoms appear at times of rest, especially in the middle of the night. "I cannot understand this" they say, "when I am busy there are no symptoms, but when I rest they come to the surface".

I explain that while they are busy, their conscious mind manages to control the activities of the body. During rest, when the conscious mind switches off, the control is released and the subconscious is allowed to express itself through physical symptoms.

Here again is a situation where the physical body is both acting to reverse an imbalance and at the same time providing a clear message as to the underlying problem.

All the symptoms given above could provide the individual with the opportunity for rest and to review their life. However, commonly they are seen as aggravations and a disruption to their busy life leading to frustration and anger. The message of the disease is lost.

Base chakra problems and insecurity are common amongst the human race and reveal our animal instincts. To feel secure on earth we need to know that we are all unique, needed and that our specific position upon the planet cannot be challenged. In knowing this we need to recognise the same in the drunk in the gutter, the murderer, the refugee and the king. Whether we can see their worth is not for us to judge as we all come from the One Source.

As we complete the link between the crown and base chakras, the physical body and the emotions are once again under the control of the Soul. This increases the awareness of one's own inner path, bringing confidence and peace.

To enable the spiritual energy to be grounded, involvement with activities linking the hands and feet to the brain are encouraged eg. gardening, painting, cooking, pottery, woodwork, walking and dancing.

The Emotions

Fear is a healthy emotion as long as it is recognised as a warning sign and not as a state of being. As a child I learnt that fire will burn. However this does not mean that every time I see a fire I panic. I have a healthy respect for the danger and can still enjoy sitting in front of a blazing fire on a cold winter's night.

Irrational fear can lead to immobilisation and paralysis and can conceal a deeper issue which the individual is unwilling to face. The letters F.E.A.R. can be seen to represent the phrase "False Expectations of an Altered Reality". Here, fear relates to an imagined problem rather than to the truth.

As inner strength and courage grow, and there is less reliance on external support, irrational fears start to dissolve and positive movement returns. The word courage comes from the French word "coeur" which means "of the heart". This says that when we come from the heart of our soul, then we will obtain courage.

The need to wear a suit of armour, to surround oneself with a thick wall or to protect oneself obsessively from outside forces reveals the level of fear. Love is the only protection we need; for only love, both of ourselves and of others, can give us total security and harmony.

Body Language

The base chakra encompasses the sacrum, the coccyx and the anal, urethral and vaginal openings. When someone is insecure or feels afraid it is common to see these areas protected either with the hands or the legs.

Some women can wind one leg several times around the other whilst both standing and sitting. Apart from doing little for the ligaments and joints, it reveals quite a deep level of insecurity and lack of trust. I find that such people are often defensive and resistant to new ideas which may shake their already unsteady environment.

Other base chakra imbalances are seen in those who cannot stand or sit still without fidgeting continuously. It is as though they feel they have no right to be here and to stand firm upon the earth.

Areas of excess adipose tissue (or fat) express a need to protect an area. Large buttocks express a desire to protect one's insecurity whilst large legs, especially in a woman, give ballast to someone who really does not want to be here, reflecting their basic insecurity and sensitivity.

Some Examples of Disharmony within the Base Chakra

1) Constipation

Rectal constipation is seen in someone who is always busy and under stress, allowing insufficient time for bodily functions. The messages of the physical body are ignored with the result that their bowels always feel "under pressure".

Such people carry excess baggage adding to their burdens instead of allowing time to release that which is no longer needed.

Another type of constipation relates to the type of person who always likes to appear in control. They hate to release their "emotions" openly and this manifests physically as a problem in releasing their "motions" or stools.

As children, we only have two ways of exerting our power over our parents: refusal of food and withholding our motions. These methods may be taken into adulthood even though their impact is focused less on others and more on the ability to remain in control.

This fear of "letting go" can be turned into an advantage. These stored emotions contain past grievances and sorrows. While they remain in the body, and are not eliminated, they can be regurgitated now and again to remind oneself just how bad things really were. Such constipated clients can give detailed accounts of events which took place over thirty years ago. It is as if their security comes from the fact that this information could be held against those who have caused harm. They love to recount their stories and feel quite aggrieved when they are told to forgive and forget!

2) Piles

Piles are blood vessels which become distended during straining and which are not given adequate time to empty before the end of defaecation.

This is often seen in the mother who is constantly disturbed, even in the toilet, by enquiring little voices allowing her little time for herself.

They are also seen in men who seek refuge to read the paper in the quietest room in the house. Suddenly they realise that time has passed and that they need to hurry, allowing insufficient time for relaxation of the system, after the act of defaecation.

Both need to learn to give time for their own bodily needs and not be ruled by the clock or the desires of others.

3) Colitis

This is an inflammatory bowel disease affecting variable lengths of the inner layer of the colon. The mucous membrane is inflamed, bleeding and ulcerated with the commonest symptom being bloody diarrhoea.

The disease can cause weakness, anaemia and pain and certainly disrupts the normal life pattern of the individual.

Hypersensitivity to certain foods is high on the list of possible causes of the disease, along with viruses and stress. This last cause must be considered for these people are often sensitive and over-react to many situations.

They are commonly perfectionists and have a fear of failure, often coming from a family where there were high expectations of achievement.

To avoid failure and their own fears, they attempt to run away which is symbolised by the diarrhoea. The process is fairly destructive and there is a level of despair in their lives. They have a fear of stopping and looking at the situation, for it is important that they are always seen to be busy (even if it is back and forth to the toilet!).

These patients need to be advised to stop running and stand still long enough to face the truth. They need loving encouragement and support as they attempt to build up their inner security.

4) Diarrhoea

Simple diarrhoea, apart from that caused by food poisoning, often occurs prior to an event as part of the anxiety symptoms.

As discussed, this is common in someone who outwardly appears in control, but inwardly is insecure about their own position in society.

They, too, need to be encouraged to stand still and to believe in their own inner strengths. It is important to remember that those who are causing the anxiety such as examiners, interviewers, audiences, etc. are also human.

5) Crohn's Disease
This is another inflammatory bowel disease involving all the layers of the gut and can occur anywhere from mouth to anus. The main symptoms are diarrhoea, pain, malabsorption and fistula formation (where channels appear between one organ and another).

Hypersensitivity to foods and viruses have once again been isolated as possible causes.

Psychospiritually, people who manifest this disease are also perfectionists, obsessive about cleanliness, achieving and "doing things right". Unlike the people with colitis, however, there is less fear and more anger which is expressed within the ball of inflammation (granuloma) which is characteristic of this disease.

Here the advice would be to "loosen up", to become more flexible and less rigid in their approach. Release the stored up anger and move forward.

All diseases of the alimentary tract are also connected with the throat chakra. This centre is related to "my will versus thy will" and many of these issues are connected with a strong or weak will. The fact that they are in the area of the base chakra links them with the desire to be perfect. Other aspects of will are met in different parts of the body and reflect a different driving force.

6) Cold Fingers and Toes
When an individual feels threatened by the environment the instinct is to withdraw into "the shell", which leaves the extremities starved of the flow of the total life force. Total self-awareness and release of fear increases the outer and inner warmth.

7) Frequency of Micturition (passing water too frequently)

This is seen in overactive individuals who are always "on the go" with the need to find the toilet at regular intervals. They know the location of all the toilets along their journey (and probably many more just in case of emergencies). Their bladder is just as overactive as they are and has a small capacity for urine before it needs to be emptied.

These individuals are usually unable to take on too much extra pressure due to the fact that their life is already overburdened with stress.

On many occasions this problem is used subconsciously to avoid the very situation which causes the stress, namely placing themselves in a position of insecurity: "I cannot come on the coach trip because there are no toilets".

8) Osteoarthrosis of the Hip

Osteoarthrosis pathologically presents with stiffness, limited movement and pain. (When there is inflammation the condition becomes osteoarth**ritis**.)

Hips are the means of moving forward or standing firm and securely upon the ground.

This disease is related to a paralysis of movement through fear of leaving that which is safe and secure. There is stiffness of the mind which holds on stubbornly to old ideas and principles. Those who present with this problem need encouragement to move forward again, one step at a time.

This usually involves changes in attitude, exercise patterns and diet. The latter is particularly important as osteoarthrosis is commonly associated with a poor diet with weight gain, which leads to further problems.

I remember going to see an old lady at home who was housebound due to arthrosis. She had told me previously that she rarely ate sweets and that her diet was wholesome. At the side of her seat was a stack of sweets and chocolates.

When questioned she told me that these were from her family who felt she needed cheering up. She did not want to hurt their feelings and so she dutifully ate through the pile before they returned home in the evening.

After a discreet word with the family, I managed to persuade them to leave fruit rather than sweets. After a month she had lost a stone in weight and was able to move more freely around her home.

Weight loss is essential for those whose arthrosis involves weight bearing joints, such as the hips and knees, and those who are overweight.

9) Kidney Stones

A stone is a collection of matter which for some reason has not been eliminated in the normal fashion. In the renal tract this can appear in any site from the kidney to the urethra and is more common where there is prolonged stress and therefore a reduction in activity of the renal muscles.

Esoterically, the elimination of fear is commonly related to the renal tract. Renal stones represent a collection of unexpressed fear in someone who outwardly appears confident but inwardly feels insecure and anxious in some area of their life.

Such people need help to express, and hence eliminate, this fear by becoming aware of their own inner security and the ability to walk freely upon their own path.

10) Hypertension

Blood pressure is the pressure exerted by the blood on the vessel walls during systole (contraction of the ventricles of the heart) and during diastole (relaxation of the ventricles). The top figure given in a reading relates to systole ... the outward pressure, and the lower figure to diastole ... the relaxing. The normal systolic blood pressure reading is 120 mm of mercury and that during diastole is 80 mm of mercury.

As doctors, we are more concerned by a raised level of diastolic blood pressure as this reflects the inability of the heart and the blood vessels to relax completely.

High blood pressure is said to be present when the diastolic reading is over 90 mm mercury, although it is not clear whether treatment should be started before the level reaches 105 mm of mercury.

Esoterically, the failure to relax fully even during an apparent rest period, shows that the individual is not able to express themselves openly and may well be hiding something from the rest of the world.

What they hide does not have to be sensational although I have had patients tell me deep personal secrets which have been hidden for a long time.

More commonly, there is an inability to be oneself for fear of not being perfect in the eyes of others. They have to be constantly alert to any detection of their insecurities and have strong issues around control.

Interestingly, many such patients are only found to have hypertension when they have a stroke which can lead to loss of control and revelation of the helpless child within.

Hardening of the arteries (arteriosclerosis) found in these patients is caused by cholesterol which comes both from the diet and is also manufactured by the liver during times of stress. It leads to inflexibility of the blood vessels which relates to the mental security through control.

To be able to talk freely and to relax has already been shown to lower the blood pressure and such techniques should be an integral part of all cardiac clinics.

11) Hypotension

Here the blood pressure levels are low, with a systolic pressure below 90 mm of mercury and diastolic below 60 mm of mercury. As has already been mentioned in previous paragraphs there is little soul pressure on the body, with the individual living a life which adapts to the needs of others rather than to their own inner requirements.

Such individuals need encouragement to bring their own energies down to earth and walk firmly along their path.

12) Impotence

The external sexual organs, such as the penis and the clitoris, are under the control of the base chakra. They can be excited without recourse to a relationship and activate the fire energy from the base of the spine.

Such energy is often experienced at an early age, long before the secondary sexual characteristics come into play. The sexual act however is not the only means of arousing the "snake" from its slumbers in the base chakra culminating in a crown chakra orgasm; many experiences can create a similar movement of energy if the individual gives himself permission to enjoy life.

Impotence, or powerlessness, commonly occurs where there is either too tight a control of the feelings or when there is such a low level of self-worth (solar plexus) that the individual must fail in this as well. The more he fails, the more he believes that he will fail.

So much emphasis has been placed on the sexual act in relation to masculinity that it is not surprising in this competitive world that impotence is on the increase. If all "the eggs are placed in one basket" and self-worth depends on the sexual act, then it reveals a desperate man.

Pride in oneself on all levels and the ability to be imperfect helps the individual to create a more balanced view of their achievements. Nobody else can give us that self worth ... it can only come from within.

13) Vaginismus

This is a condition where the vaginal muscles are so tight that they prevent intercourse or at least cause it to be extremely uncomfortable.

There are many different causes although the commonest seen is related to sexual abuse during childhood and/or adolescence. The powerlessness experienced causes the individual to exert all the power they do possess in attempting to close the place of entry.

Abuse is linked with the sacral and throat chakras and becomes embroiled with fear to express oneself and guilt at what has happened. In many cases the individual protects themself by switching off the sexual desire and creating numbness around the pelvic area.

These women need specialised counselling and a caring partner who is secure in their own right and can allow the power of the sexual act to be equally distributed between the two participants.

14) Congenital Structural Changes to the Feet

The feet are the site through which spirit meets matter. When I see someone whose sole of the foot is turned away from the earth (club foot) or is raised high above it (pes cavus), then I find myself facing a very sensitive soul who is not sure if they want to come down onto this earth.

There is commonly fear and insecurity which even manifests at their birth with a long, difficult labour, breathing problems or overdue in dates. Their reluctance to arrive may be followed by protests in the first few years of life, ie. crying, temper tantrums or physical problems.

Such children need firm but loving support with encouragement to stay the course. It may be not until the age of 28 years (their first Saturn return), that they start to allow the soul energy to enter their body and make some imprint on the earth's surface.

Suggestions to Balance the Activity of the Base Chakra

1) Do not be too proud and controlled to recognise there is a problem. See that what you do not like in others is a reflection of your own inner being, trying to be heard.

2) Put away the stick which strikes you every time you are not perfect ... stop giving yourself a hard time. Love yourself.

3) Be glad that you are imperfect and that you make mistakes. Perfection is not balanced. Balance is achieved by accepting the perfect and imperfect parts of your nature.

4) Recognise your uniqueness and that with this knowledge there is no place for personal competition. Soul pressure will maintain the stress we need to move forward.

5) Choose relaxing pastimes which are not setting time against space, e.g. 20 lengths of the swimming pool in 10 minutes induces strain. Choose a goal from either time or space, not both.

6) Make your own decision to stay on earth and to enjoy life.

This does not mean that there will not be hard times, but they are much easier to handle with the help of the full soul pressure rather than while you are partially out of your body.

7) Good grounding exercises are those involving the garden, the kitchen, pottery, art and walking. Stand, if possible, on the earth without shoes and feel the earth energies pull your feet towards the centre of the planet.

8) Choose the colour red when selecting items of clothing which involve the base chakra and which will enhance any grounding exercises, eg. shoes, trousers, socks, skirts etc.

Remember that too much red can create quite an energy in the base and therefore alternate with deeper shades of red or other colours when well grounded.

9) Lean against a tree and feel the strength of the tree which has probably been on earth for many hundreds of years. Allow your feet to feel like the roots of the tree, passing deep within the ground, and imagine your own head and arms stretching up towards the light, realigning base and crown chakras.

10) Do something which is fun and allows your inner child to play. Once again, this is best if it involves earth or water but may be something which was always forbidden at home and therefore suppressed in the attempt to "be perfect".

11) Stand firm upon the ground with the knees slightly bent and say; "I have a unique place here on earth and, in that knowledge, I can feel secure".

Chapter 8

The Sacral Chakra

THE SACRAL CHAKRA	
Position	: Lower Abdomen
Spiritual Aspect	: Self-Respect
Basic Need	: Creativity within Relationships
Related Emotions	: Possessiveness, Sharing
Endocrine Glands	: Ovaries and Testes
Associated Organs	: Uterus, Large Bowel, Prostate, Ovaries, Testes
Colour	: Orange

Anatomy of the Ovaries/Testes

In the foetus the testes or ovaries develop in the lower abdomen; the former descending to the scrotum by birth. Here the production of the sperm can be carried out at temperatures slightly lower than those of the rest of the body.

Esoterically, the etheric link to the testes, is formed during gestation and therefore comes from the sacral chakra.

Physiology of the Sex Glands

The nucleus of the cells of the male contains XY chromosomes and that of the female XX chromosomes. These provide the basic anatomical and physiological identity to the different genders.

At puberty, the female's ovaries start to secrete their hormones **oestrogen and progesterone** and in the male the testes start to produce their hormone **testosterone**.

These hormones act on the anatomy, the physiology and the

psychology of the individual to produce secondary sexual characteristics.

The Link Between Spiritual and Physical Creation

The eggs of the ovaries and the sperm of the testes represent the seeds which will guarantee the continuation of the human race. Within this knowledge, it could be said that the eggs and sperm carry the creative life force which is passed down from matter itself.

During sexual intercourse, energy relating to spirit is released from the base chakra and enters matter. This interaction between spirit/father and matter/mother leads to the creation of the son/soul whose role is ultimately to guarantee the continuation of life.

This pattern is repeated wherever there is an interaction between two opposite poles, ie. spirit and matter, male and female, dominant and recessive, yin and yang, with the creation of a third party which preserves the essence of the original partnership but where the new form is at a higher level of consciousness.

This is the purpose behind all relationships, ie. that we should not only find ourselves but, in doing this, also create something which is greater than the sum of the parts. In this way the original Source of all Life is continually growing showing that nothing in this universe is static.

Following the fertilisation of the egg by the sperm (which is symbolic of the spiritual interaction), a single celled zygote is formed. Within minutes this cell has divided and multiplied to create a multicellular form. This process is symbolic of the many divisions of the original soul.

For man, the gestation period is nine months during which time there will be a deepening of the relationship between spirit and matter. Common bonds are formed which act as the means of communication between the two poles of the partnership. Such bonds are essential for the life force to flow. Without them, there is death. The words common, communication, community all come from a similar source which means "belonging equally to". To find this equality in a relationship needs self-respect and respect for the partner. This is the spiritual aspect of the sacral chakra.

At birth, the strong links with the Source are lost but the interaction between spirit and matter are deeply ingrained in the inner being. Following their lead, the individual follows a path towards self-consciousness by seeking out those parts of himself which are not fully revealed.

This is achieved by connecting with others on the planet and seeing a reflection of ourselves in the mirror which they provide. Sometimes we like what we see and at other times we shy away from the truth.

Relationships

Any significant relationship holds a key to open a door to part of ourselves which is hidden. By recognising, accepting and loving this part, we can achieve wholeness and health.

We cannot hope to find all that we seek in one person for the only place that our shadow side exists is within. We all possess a "soul-mate" who is identical and who was formed at the same time as ourselves. To meet your soul-mate is extremely rare for to have two people doing the same work, in the same place, is a waste of valuable resources. To marry such a "twin" would lead to stagnation of growth.

It is more likely that, when we feel closely connected to someone, they are of the same soul-group which means there is a common thread linking the group's purpose on earth.

It is more common to find small parts of ourselves in many people. When we realise this we will become more lenient with our partner from whom we expect the world and often feel disappointed when their performance does not live up to our expectations!

Relationships come in all shapes and sizes:

a) We are connected to our family through blood ties. These are very strong even though there may be little else in common.

b) We can feel a very strong attraction to someone whom we met in previous lives and where there is unfinished business.

Outwardly there may be little in common but the pull cannot be resisted.

c) We relate easily to those people with whom we consciously detect a common link. They validate our beliefs and help us to feel secure.

A common link provides a line of communication for any relationship. The link does not have to be positive, ie. two people may be bonded by their hatred for each other. Such a bond may tie them physically more tightly than if it were a bond of love.

d) We relate less easily to those with whom there is an unconscious link. That which irritates us in others, is often present in ourselves. It is important to see our world as a place of learning. Everybody has a message to help us along our soul path.

For example:
I feel irritated by the aggressive nature of my boss.
He makes me feel small and insignificant.
He criticises me in front of others. I want to tell him what I think, but don't feel strong enough.
My boss is expressing his own insecurity through his aggressive behaviour. My insecurity prevents me from acting. We both have an imbalance within the base chakra reflecting a lack of inner strength.

e) Relationships can be strained between ourselves and those who are able to express something which we find difficult. eg. the girl who cries at the slightest pressure, attracting sympathy, annoys the strong capable type who would secretly like the attention but is frightened of becoming vulnerable. There is a lesson to be learnt.

f) At other times, we are attracted to those who have an attitude or feature which we admire. In most cases this is showing us that this same aspect is present inside ourselves if we only know where to look.

g) We are attracted to a member of the opposite sex who has characteristics which represent our own "shadow gender". We are all both male and female, despite outward appearances, and it is the search for the "other half" which in many cases leads us into a relationship.

The soul is androgynous and it is this state which we are working towards; not through suppression of either our masculinity or femininity, but through the union of both to create a new combined form.

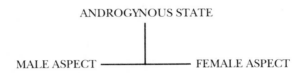

ANDROGYNOUS STATE

MALE ASPECT ——————— FEMALE ASPECT

g) We are often attracted to someone who can satisfy areas of our life in which we feel deficient. This may mean that we marry someone who has the money, the intelligence or the family which are absent in our own life.

Or we may look for someone who is strong and on whom we can depend. Or we may choose someone who has a spiritual awareness which we feel we lack.

Many relationships are symbiotic, mutually rewarding, each contributing where the other is deficient. Unfortunately, this comfortable state of affairs may stagnate soul growth as there is no need for either to strive for their individual self-awareness. On the death of a partner, the person who remains may be left unable to cope without the assistance of their "other half". Their grief may lead to an early grave, literally dying of a broken heart.

In other cases, the death allows the remaining partner to start to live their life from their own inner being and they find strengths which they never knew they possessed.

The perfect relationship is one built on love, respect and honesty where both partners are able to remain whole and yet be enhanced by the union.

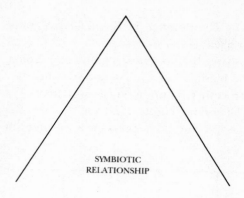

SYMBIOTIC
RELATIONSHIP

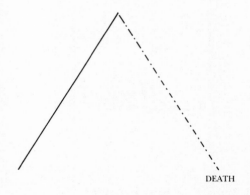

DEATH

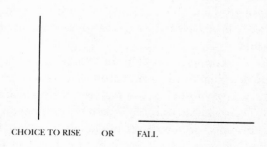

CHOICE TO RISE   OR   FALL.

As spoken by The Prophet (by Kahlil Gibran) when talking about marriage:
Give your hearts, but not into each other's keeping.
For only the hand of Life can contain your hearts.
And stand together yet not too near together:
For the pillars of the temple stand apart,
And the oak tree and the cypress grow not in each other's shadow."

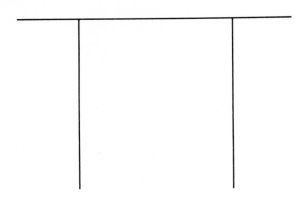

BALANCED RELATIONSHIP

Spiritual Aspect ... Self Respect

Self-respect means to give space to our creative impulses so that a true union between spirit and matter can occur. Without this we cannot grow and this can lead to resentment towards those whom we believe have hampered the development of our own inner child.

Abuse is a common problem in society today whether it is emotional, sexual or physical. It comes from a lack of respect for the needs of another but ultimately reflects a lack of respect for self. The cycle can only be broken by building up a level of inner self-respect which meets the needs of the soul and not the self-fulfilling prophecy of the personality. This is difficult for a child to achieve alone and they therefore require love, support and guidance from those who can stand back from their own personal needs.

The fine balance between interdependence and independence, which is the goal in any relationship, depends on the recognition, respect and love shown towards the spiritual essence within both parties.

One of the most important means of maintaining a level of respect is through the power of communication (the common bond); without this the relationship is bound to die. It may mean that through communication the two partners may wish to part, but even this can be mutually beneficial if it occurs through common agreement.

An analogy

There were two porcupines living in the Arctic. It was very cold and they decided to huddle close together to stay warm. As they came closer, their needle-shape spines started to injure the other's skin. They moved apart and became cold. They moved closer and felt pain.

They spent many months before they found the right balance. Close enough to give warmth but not too close to cause pain.

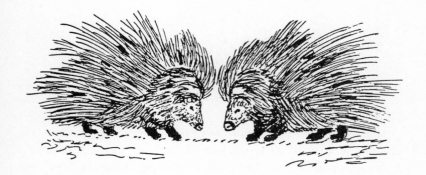

The Emotions

The sacral chakra is related to space and boundaries. A mother's womb provides a warm and supportive framework while at the same time having the capability to expand its size in order to accommodate the growth of the baby.

Such flexibility whilst maintaining one's own boundaries is essential for any relationship.

Too little space can lead to cramped development and can be caused by a partner who is possessive, clingy and dependent. Their underlying problem is insecurity surrounding poor self-worth. Their whole identity is often based on their role within this relationship.

This can be seen in a marriage, between parents and children or just within a friendship. Such dependence stifles the growth of both parties and can destroy the relationship. This outcome often leads to hurt and a feeling of abandonment with a fear of entering another relationship.

Hence the other pole of existence appears, ie. lack of commitment in a relationship, a strong desire to stay independent and a determination never to be hurt again.

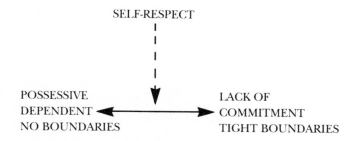

Just as the porcupines spent months perfecting the perfect balance, so too may we spend many lifetimes learning how to nurture our own inner child fully whilst respecting and accepting the needs of others.

The sacral and throat chakras are interlinked as they are both connected with creativity. The latter is often inappropriately used to express sacral chakra blocks. Hence, the frustrated housewife continually nags her husband to help with the household chores and then turns on her teenage son, whose room she describes as looking like a "rubbish tip".

Both forms of nagging are offered in the name of love although ultimately they lead to restriction of growth. When one person is providing 90% of the attention to any detail, it leaves only 10% to be contributed by the other person.

If the nagging wife pulls back to 50%, then she allows her husband to come forward. Similarly, when the teenager is left to his own devices for a while, he will eventually either tidy his room or "die" buried under a mass of clothes, magazines, sweet wrappers, dirty coffee cups, etc.!

Constant nagging is not communicating … it is one-sided and inhibits growth. Act or accept. The best relationship is one where both partners put in 100% and both get out 100% … 50% and 50% is a good start!

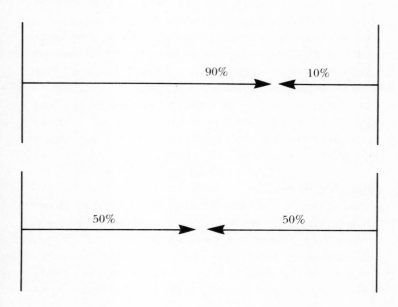

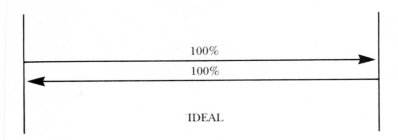

By nagging, or by spending so much time trying to change others, we are often avoiding our own issues of growth which also relate to the throat chakra. We must change ourselves before we can hope that others will change.

The umbilical cord is a very strong link between parents and children, whether male or female. When the love which flows along the cord is unconditional, then the link is pure. However, if the cord (the love) is knotted with conditions, then the tie may need to be cut before a new bond can be formed.

Such cutting can be more difficult than cutting the physical cord at birth. Many negative conditions hold a relationship together. These include guilt, fear of loneliness, fear of not being loved and fear of not being accepted.

But such ties will eventually strangle the partnership, denying both participants the life blood which they need. True love sets another free. Each can then stand apart and give unconditional love and support.

Changing Roles

In the past fifty years, the roles of men and women have changed dramatically. The World Wars proved that women could work as hard and as profitably as men. Women now work through financial need or through the need to satisfy their own desires.

In a similar way, there are more and more men sharing the responsibility for the care of the children and maintaining the house. This trend represents the equality of the sexes and the need to recognise and accept the feminine qualities within every man and the masculine qualities within every woman.

With the advent of single parent families we are starting to see the role of the nurturer and of the breadwinner being combined within one person. This may be an important step towards an androgynous state as long as the supportive energy for such a state comes from the level of the soul.

A far greater shift has taken place within human consciousness where women are learning to be more assertive and logical, and men to contact their intuitive and feeling nature. This naturally will result in the blending of the two aspects.

After years of conditioning, it is not easy to move from one pattern to another and hence there is inevitable resistance to such change, both on the part of society and on the part of the individual. This resistance often manifests within the physical body as disease.

Nowadays, I recognise that the shift may have gone too far for many career women are out of touch with their femininity and many sensitive men are finding it extremely difficult to work in a male-orientated society.

Like all swings, the roles will eventually reach a balance. The transition period will be far smoother if we learn to accept all parts of ourselves with equal importance.

Disharmony within the sacral chakra is often related to the mental driver "be strong" which leads to feelings of inadequacy, ie. not being "man enough" or "not being the ideal wife or mother". These thoughts are often based on socially preconceived ideas of what constitutes the perfect man or woman. Fortunately, times are changing fast although the "male chauvinist" and the "little housewife" are still lurking inside and may need to be acknowledged before they eventually disappear.

Body Language

Here the sensitive area is over the sacral chakra. This represents the ability to create and to be given the space for this creation. Sometimes there is a desire not to let go of the creation, leading to a possessiveness which can be seen in bloating or an increase in body fat over the lower abdomen.

In women, it is a fear of transferring their creativity from producing children to producing something from their own inner self. Many have only been someone's daughter, someone's mother or someone's wife. To be oneself can be quite frightening and therefore they hold onto that which they know.

For men, their possessiveness can be seen in terms of their family or their material possessions.

Placing the hands across the lower abdomen, may be due to etiquette or may represent a fear of being hurt or not respected. These issues need to be recognised when dealing with anybody presenting with body language relating to the sacral chakra. Safe space, linked with unconditional love, must be given to allow the individual to express themselves fully.

Some Examples of Dis-ease Related to the Sacral Chakra

1) Irritable Bowel Disease

This is an extremely common condition which is also known as "spastic colon". It can be found in both sexes although it is more common in females. The bowel itself is in perfect condition and the problem lies in an imbalance within the nervous system which supplies the gut.

Following a trigger, the bowel goes through phases of spasm giving abdominal pain, bloating and constipation, followed by release of stools and wind. This causes an imbalance in the environment of the bowel which may lead to an overgrowth of certain microbes such as "candida" or a hypersensitivity to different foods.

These secondary effects require treatment but the possible underlying psychospiritual imbalance must also be considered.

The disharmony lies in the desire to become independent (the release) whilst remaining emotionally dependent (the spasm). It is commonly found where parent/child boundaries are not clear, eg. during mother-in-law visits or when the children leave home. Those who manifest this illness are often caring, conscientious people who tend to keep their feelings inside whatever happens. They look after the needs of others before asking that their own needs will be met. However, an inner resentment often develops which literally "screws them up inside" leading to the spasms.

In the end they must choose not to react in response to the feelings of the other person but to act from a position of their own self-respect. Using their throat chakra they learn to express their needs and their feelings and realise that they are not responsible for the reactions of others.

2) Problems Relating to the Female Reproductive System

The Menstrual Cycle
There are various illnesses under this heading and each needs to be considered on its merits. However, the main feature is related to the creative flow of life as described above.

The menstrual cycle follows the pattern of creation with the first part of the cycle symbolic of the energy flowing into spirit (the egg) and the second part, after ovulation, symbolic of the reception of that egg by matter (the womb).

When there is no fertilisation, the egg and the womb lining are released (menstruation) and this "death" allows a new birth to occur as another egg is ripened. Each cycle acts to preserve and enrich the life force enhancing the energy in the sacral chakra.

A) The premenstrual syndrome is represented by irritability, clumsiness, food cravings, a desire to be alone, weeping, tender breasts and bloating and relates to disharmony in the second part of the cycle.

Whereas this should be a time for nurturing and preparing the nest, in this modern world, there is little time available for such feminine requirements, leading to confusion of identity and frustration.

This is a special time for women and, instead of comfort feeding to suppress the feminine desires, extra space should be given towards nurturing and responding to one's own sensitivity.

B) Problems of the menstrual flow
Whether the periods are too heavy or too light shows an imbalance within the feminine force within the individual. This may

have been damaged by past traumas especially where there were issues around respect.

a) **Menorrhagia** or heavy periods represents tears of frustration, as the feminine part of the individual is denied its creative expression. It is important to get in touch with the inner girl-child and to nurture and recognise her beauty.

b) **Amenorrhoea** or loss of periods can occur for a number of reasons which may be structural or hormonal.

For some women, their lack of periods occurs at a time of stress when these non-essential organs are switched off by the sympathetic nervous system.

For others, it occurs alongside other features which symbolise high levels of male hormones present in the blood, such as hairiness, weight gain, voice changes.

Such women may well have mentally disconnected their feminine side as it was not acceptable within the world in which they lived. They need encouragement and help to learn how to express their femininity and to be proud of it.

Amenorrhoea is also a feature of anorexia nervosa which is a multi-chakra problem and is discussed under the heading of diseases of the throat chakra.

C) Uterine Fibroid

This is an area of overgrowth of the muscle layer of the uterus which forms itself into a ball. Fibroids can reach a considerable size before they are noticed and most women of child-bearing age probably possess one or two fibroids.

Their presence in the muscle layer suggests a build up of tension which has not been released. The womb is the site of nurturing and they are commonly seen in women who have nurtured the growth of others to the exclusion of their own need for nurturing.

A question which usually elicits an emotional response is;

"Who nurtures you?"

There is unspoken resentment with the desire to make space within their life for their own needs especially those of their Inner Child. If the outer world is unable to provide the parenting we require, we need to look within and learn to parent ourselves.

The discovery of fibroids provides an opportunity for letting go of commitments which are no longer necessary and seeing the womb symbolically as a room where one is surrounded by those things which bring warmth and caring.

In Chinese medicine, resentment relates to disharmony in the energy fields of the liver meridian which should also be treated.

D) Ovarian Cysts

Any cyst represents hurt or pain which has not been released. The fluid in the cyst is symbolic of tears. Ovarian cysts come in all sizes, some benign and some malignant. They usually grow quietly and give insidious symptoms which can be confused with many other diseases.

When the cyst occurs in the area of the creative life force it suggests that something has happened to prevent its release.

It has been seen that many women with a cyst have been abused at some time, whether emotionally or physically. There is a feeling that their wishes are not respected along with a sensation of powerlessness.

To take back their power and self-respect and release the old hurts and pains, is very important.

E) Endometriosis

In this disease, endometrium (the lining of the womb) is found outside the womb, most commonly in the pelvis, especially around the ovaries and fallopian tubes. This means that with every period these areas also bleed, causing pain and adhesions. Why this happens is not medically known but there is evidence, on a psychological level, that many of these women had poor sex education, much of which was negative and portrayed periods as being "the curse of women".

Hopefully, there is now a more positive approach to the information given concerning the female cycle. But until women respect themselves fully these problems will still occur. Pregnancy often sends the disease into remission for many years which would validate the claim that, when a woman uses her body for the purpose for which it was meant, the negative ideas are released.

3) Problems Relating to the Male Reproductive System

A) Testicular Disease

Tumours of the testes are becoming more common. Like the ovaries, they contain the life force from which all life commences. If this is blocked for any reason then the build-up can lead to changes on a cellular level. I have seen men who were ashamed of their sexual activities and a few months later developed testicular cancers.

Once again, there has to be a balance between respect and love for others, and respect and love for oneself.

B) Prostatic Disease

The prostate gland produces some of the nourishment and fluid required for the journey of the sperm. It could be said that it mirrors the nurturing abilities of the female womb.

I believe that prostate enlargement, benign and malignant, relates to the failure to feel nurtured at an early age which later may be sought through the sexual act. But because the basic feeling is absent leaves the recipient empty and cold. The ability to allow warmth in, requires a man to surrender some of his inbuilt barriers.

60% of 60 year old men have enlargement of this gland with urinary problems and yet in the medical profession we are a long way from understanding the cause.

Exercises to Balance the Sacral Chakra

1) Choose to respect oneself. This means laying down some boundaries but giving space for creative expression.

2) Understand that within this respect is the ability to control your part in any relationship.

3) Learn to communicate, which means both speaking and hearing (involving the throat chakra). Work to find a compromise or common place of agreement from which the relationship can progress.

4) When experiencing difficulties within a relationship, sit quietly and imagine your partner sitting opposite. Now draw a triangle between you, with the third angle equidistant above

your heads. Allow the energy of your higher selves to meet at this point.

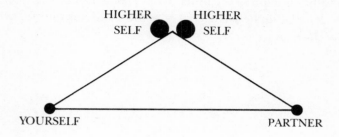

HIGHER SELF   HIGHER SELF

YOURSELF   PARTNER

The higher self is beyond the personality and can communicate with objective compassion. Ask the higher self of your partner what he/she needs from you. Tell them what you need. Attempt to find a mutually acceptable solution to your problem.

If one cannot be found then accept this and through your higher self, ask that those spiritual energies which care for your partner should come close and support him/her as you can no longer maintain this role. Wrap them in a "loving pink blanket" and let them go.

This exercise incorporates some of the ideas related to "cutting the ties which bind" which are strongly recommended to anybody who has problems in the sacral chakra. ("Cutting the Ties that Bind" by Phyllis Krystal.)

5) Use the colour orange to bring the energies of this area into life. The colour blue, from the throat chakra, can also be used to enable one to express the feelings from within the sacral chakra.

6) Using creative visualisation, see people or animals which represent your masculine and feminine parts. Observe their features and what they have to say to you. Work at finding a common bond which may be represented by a third person or animal. Recognise and acknowledge their assets.

7) Accept and appreciate both the masculine and feminine parts of yourself. Allow the inner children to play. Nurture and worship the woman inside with oils, baths, scents, clothes, etc.; allow the strength of the inner man to come forth.

8) Recognise the sacral chakra as the womb for the creativity of the soul.

Chapter 9

The Solar Plexus Chakra

THE SOLAR PLEXUS CHAKRA	
Position	: Epigastrium, Below the Ribs
Spiritual Aspect	: Self-Worth
Basic Need	: Valuing the Needs of the Self
Related Emotions	: Anger, Resentment, Unworthiness, Guilt
Endocrine Gland	: Pancreas
Associated Organs	: Liver, Spleen, Stomach, Small Intestine
Colour	: Yellow

The Anatomy of the Pancreas

The pancreas is situated beneath the stomach with its head supported by the curve of the duodenum. The liver and gall bladder are lateral to its head in the right hypochondrium, while the spleen is lateral to its tail, in the left hypochondrium.

The Physiology of the Pancreas

The pancreas produces the hormones **insulin, glucagon and somatostatin** from its endocrine glands and **digestive enzymes** from its exocrine glands.

Insulin is essential for the uptake of glucose into the cells where it is used as an energy source for most of the activities of the cell. Insulin also enables glucose to be stored in the liver and the muscles as **glycogen**. During stress, this glucose is released into the blood stream under the influence of

adrenaline and cortisone. These hormones therefore antago-
nise the action of insulin.

The Power of Attraction

The heart chakra and the solar plexus are the centres of desire,
responding to the energies which emerge from the Astral or
emotional body. While the dominant influence on our life is
to meet the needs of the personality, there will be little energy
passing through the heart chakra, the majority moving down
to the solar plexus.

However, as soul consciousness expands, there is an increase
in the energy emerging from the heart chakra and a reduction
in that through the lower chakra.

The solar plexus acting like the sun, attracts towards it all
that is needed to complete the process of creation which was
started in the base and sacral chakras. When all the "ingredients" are brought together they are transformed, turning the
energy into something which meets the needs of the personality. In physical terms this is called **assimilation**.

The sun emits an electro-magnetic force which provides light
and heat; the light is an attracting force whilst the heat acts as
a transformer.

Glucose, as a source of energy, is the key to creating that
transforming potential within the physical body. It enables us
to survive, regenerate and, hence, to grow.

The Seat of the Emotions

The desires of the personality are met by converting the energy
of an idea into an emotion and then allowing this to be
expressed. The emotion acts as a magnet, attracting towards it
that which we desire; we feel happy, we attract happiness.
Unfortunately, the desires of the personality are often linked
with expectations and conditions and, although some of these
may be met, we also have to accommodate other features which
may not be so welcome, ie. "I'll be happy as long as it does not
rain" can lead to long periods of unhappiness in an English cli-
mate!

Expressing an impulse, without conditions, frees one to

enjoy life to the fullest and to live totally in the present, ie. "I am happy".

The solar plexus could therefore be said to be the seat of the emotions. It is the area in which we find the ego (with a small "e") and relates to personal power or self-worth.

In many spiritual groups great strides are made to defeat the ego and to eradicate it from one's being. However, the force sent to fight it is none other than the ego itself, in the form of the personality, and it soon becomes clear that such a battle is lost before it starts.

We need an ego. It is the vehicle for the desires of the soul. Our ego allows us to walk firmly and with confidence along the path. Without it, we hide all that we are behind a bushel, wasting a valuable incarnation.

The solar plexus is the site of conditional love while the heart relates to unconditional love. The personality lays down the conditions in order to maintain its hold on the individual. If the personality can be shown that it is needed and useful, it is more likely to agree to work under the guidance of the soul than when it is threatened with destruction. It can then start to release its conditions on the gift of love and begin to trust in a Higher Power.

The Spiritual Attribute ... Self-Worth

Self-worth is the ability to value oneself for just "being you". The next stage, which relates to the heart chakra, is to love oneself. The two are closely linked, although the pathway to the latter is through the former.

In this world of duality, inner self-worth comes through valuations in the outer world, which after a while no longer hold any importance. This does not mean that we do not enjoy praise or attention but that we are no longer dependent upon it for our self-image.

First, therefore, we need to experience external valuations which are easily found as the main content in any small talk:

"How do you do?" "Who are you?" "What do you do?" "Are you married; do you have children?", etc.

An identity based on external criteria.

The personality needs to reinforce its self-worth and therefore attracts towards it that which will satisfy its needs. This means it will look for praise, attention, adoration and may only feel content with its performance when it receives these from an external audience.

The goal of the personality is to believe in itself without this audience. This is not selfish or self-centred but fully accepting all that we are with an internal pride.

To deny all that we are is to deny our Creator.

Once this has been established, the next step is to recognise the desires of the soul and to move the attracting force from the needs of the personality to those of the soul. This transformation takes the energy of the solar plexus into the heart chakra.

As we move along this path, we meet two poles of existence within the astral field which relate to self-worth. One is "the pleaser" whose identity is totally dependent on the ability to please others and to be needed by others. The other is the "selfish individual" who appears very self-contained and self-assured.

In essence there is no separation; they are two points around a central focus. Both have poor self-worth, but one manages to hide it better than the other. When working at the solar plexus level we may swing from one stage to the other or may stay rigidly within one camp, terrified of allowing the shadow side to show.

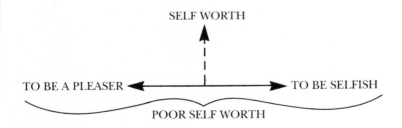

Little do we realise that the shadow is very obvious to everybody except ourselves and that despite the shadow we are still loved.

The pleaser is terrified of becoming selfish but, as has been shown previously, their constant need for re-assurance, attention and love leads to a state which can be very self-centred and manipulative.

Manipulation is something which is found in all three of the dominant chakras (the base, the solar plexus and the throat), where there are major issues around control. Most manipulation is subtle, laced with charm, and usually appears on an emotional level:

"Nobody comes to see me" after the family has visited twice a day.

"I know I'm not important and that you have more interesting people to visit".

"Don't worry; it only took me four hours to prepare the meal; I can understand if work comes first".

"I have been ill with worry; you did not ring me all day?" When asked why they did not ring to find out what had happened the reply is: "I did not want to bother you".

All these comments, with shades of emotional blackmail, verge on the "martyr syndrome" which is an image commonly found within the solar plexus and is guaranteed to incite guilt in the listener if they have any unfinished business in their own solar plexus.

The martyr says:

"To be worthy of my place in society, I must suffer".

"I must not complain" which often represents deep rooted religious teachings and family standards.

"We are here to suffer, not to enjoy life".

The "cross" is rarely laid down and, indeed, there is utter consternation if one offers to ease their burden by carrying the cross for a short while.

The pleaser's initial desire is to care for another person, which is an admirable ambition and one with which I am myself involved. However, when the carer's identity and self-worth is dependent on "being needed", then conditions are placed on the caring which can seriously affect the quality of help offered.

Giving and receiving unconditional love is not simple. However kind-hearted, it is not easy to release all interest in your gift once it has been offered.

As a therapist, when the client returns for their next visit, the immediate question is:

"How are you"?

If there is poor self-worth, then the answer "No better" does little for one's confidence. The immediate thought may be:

"It is all their fault. If only they had done as I told them".

This can be followed by either:

"I knew they would not change, I'll ask them to leave".

Or "That's it; I'll close my practice and become a lotus eater!"

It is just the same within the home when someone has to ask for comments on their work or question the level of loving. The answer rarely enhances confidence and in many cases makes it worse as they feel guilty for having asked in the first place.

"Do I look nice?" to a tired over-worked husband.

"Yes dear, you always look lovely; is dinner ready?"

Then there are the debts which need to be paid. It is as if, following the act of giving, a fishing line was cast; the hook catches just in time to remind the receiver that, although on one level the gift was free, on another there is a debt to pay.

"After all I did for you, is this the way you repay me?"

"They never thanked me for that present I sent ... some people have no manners".

"I was always there for them; where were they when I needed them?"

It is very difficult to explain to such a caring person that they have no right to expect anything in return. Any expectation reveals that their caring was tinged with conditions. Such hooks can lead to resentment and anger at the way in which the individual has been treated. Unfortunately, the pleaser, who still wants to be liked, is fearful of letting out this resentment in case it leads to a scene or splits the family.

The fact that nobody is talking in the family or that when they do it is in cutting tones, with snide remarks, has little to do with the issue. The anger builds within the mind and starts to pollute the level of care which is being offered.

For example:

The daughter goes to visit her house-bound mother as a duty rather than a desire. She shouts at her mother who is not ready for their outing, banging the wheelchair down the stairs.

At the end of the visit the old lady is exhausted and the daughter frustrated.

Neither can benefit from such a visit. It is offered for the wrong reasons and therefore is bound to fail. Once again communication is the key to the problem. But, if this has been lacking for many years, it is not easy to start the ball rolling.

At this stage the victim and the victimiser come into play. Both parties feel victimised and neither is willing to break the cycle and "rescue" the situation. Status quo exists.

Only by owning one's feelings and choosing whether that which is being offered belongs to you can the process start to move forward again. There may need to be some tears and some anger but these should be offered into the centre of the discussion and not directed at anyone in particular by saying "I feel angry" rather than "You make me angry".

Nobody **makes** us do anything unless **we choose** to play the victim. It is the inability to say "no" for fear of being rejected that leads to many continuing their pattern of pleasing.

"I don't want to let others down (even though it is inconvenient and I am exhausted)". The job is done but not always with good grace.

There are some who end up like door-mats with little self-respect due to poor levels of self-worth and an eagerness to please.

The day that they do say "no" everybody raises their hands in horror; "how could she let us down after 20 years on the white elephant stall". Guilt is piled upon the pleaser who almost gives in and returns to the stall. But if time is allowed to pass someone else is chosen to take her place and her name is quickly forgotten.

This, of course, is one of the worries of the pleaser that someone else can do the job as well as they can. They need to be needed and hence will deny any illness or weakness rather than give in. They are the "copers"; those who, when asked "How are you?", will always answer "I'm fine", despite pain and suffering. They are conscientious workers and "good little boys and girls".

Their role as a carer can lead to co-dependency problems where their addiction for caring brings them into contact with those who are addicted to other means of enhancing their self-worth, such as alcohol, gambling and drugs.

The carer always believes that someday their addicted partner will change and tries harder to please. Breaking the cycle needs courage and the realisation that things are out of control.

There are many co-dependency support groups now in existence, emphasising the widespread problem. Caring is a noble cause and therefore often missed as a form of addiction. We are all addicted to something in differing degrees (alcohol, gambling, drugs, work, caring, etc.); the criteria for the need for help is measured on the degree of dependency. Unfortunately, it is not always easy to be objective about one's own form of addiction.

When there is an eagerness to please, then the solar plexus is wide open and can act as a sponge for any energies which are in the vicinity.

Such people often find themselves exhausted by the end of the day having picked up a variety of negative and positive energies as well as being drained by "human vultures". This commonly occurs in the caring professions when the clients feel refreshed and the therapist is drained. One of the purposes of sitting behind a desk, or wearing a white coat, is that they provide some cover for the leaking of energy from the solar plexus.

The more stressed the individual, the more eager to please and the more exhausted they become. Eventually "burn-out" occurs which can involve both the throat and base chakras. Here, the nurturing needs to be reversed and time is needed to repair the damage.

The pleaser is extremely sensitive to comments concerning them and can become paranoid concerning the thoughts belonging to others. The desire to please can lead to a chameleon-like existence where the sensitivity of the solar plexus is used to detect that which is required to please the audience. This is a dangerous game to play as it can mean that the individual loses themselves along the way. There are many people who play this game sub-consciously and are totally out of touch with their own inner truth.

Sensitivity to others leads to an inability for some individuals to enter an environment where the energies are mildly out of alignment. This is usually seen in those whose psychic talents are well developed and where the solar plexus is used as an antennae to transmit these subtle energies.

They can become quite anxious within an unstable environment or when sitting next to someone whose energies are unsettled. Such people need to be shown how to protect or close this centre and to rely on their intuition, through the heart and crown chakras, rather than on their "gut feelings" from the solar plexus.

At the other end of the spectrum is someone who appears selfish, always looking after their own needs before those of others. I have found that this is an acquired act built upon many years of inadequacy and poor confidence. On many occasions alcohol helps to boost the confidence and it becomes part of the daily routine.

It is very difficult to break down the defences which have been built to protect a vulnerable inner core and can only be achieved by enhancing the inner confidences, so that the individual feels safe enough to remove the wall with their own hands.

Someone who is truly confident of their own self-worth does not have to tell everybody. They can sell themselves clearly and objectively. The need to boast or blow one's own trumpet reveals an ailing confidence needing reassurance and support.

Poor self-worth can mean that it is difficult to ask for help or to ask that your needs are met. Such requests signify a level of failure and weakness and hence things tend to be kept inside. These people are non-complainers; they will suffer all levels of abuse rather than "hurt others". They can carry tremendous burdens of guilt which they handle manfully rather than face up to their oppressor. They avoid conflict at any cost and can be seen to be the peace-maker.

In the end, there is a constant battle between the pleaser and the one who resents being used:

"He makes me so mad, but I do not want to say anything as he is so moody".

"I resent the way in which she uses me, but I do not want to cause her any upset".

Until the pleaser decides to speak out, and risk an upset, the situation will continue. On most occasions, the reactions are no worse than the original stalemate.

Those with poor self-worth can become listeners. They listen but do not talk because they feel they have nothing to say; they don't want to bother people and have a fear that nobody will listen. However, when they are given the space to talk, they cannot be stopped and may go on regardless of the needs of the other person. Now, the new listener has to make a stand, reflecting their own self-worth by setting limits on the time and energy given to this person at one sitting.

It is not uncommon to hear that the same procedure has been repeated several times, and that on each occasion the new listener was told that they were the only one to be trusted which, of course, can always boost an ailing ego.

Body Language

The solar plexus is the most common chakra to need protection, as it is through this area that one can pick up vibrational changes in the atmosphere, especially those emanating from the emotional planes.

Crossing the hands over the stomach may represent someone who is cold, but this action is more significant when it occurs sub-consciously when sensitive questions are asked. It reveals a sensitivity to issues around self-worth and a need to protect oneself from further pain.

As stated earlier, sitting behind a desk conveniently covers the solar plexus. If you want an honest conversation with someone ask them to come round the desk and talk to you face to face.

A large "beer belly" covers the solar plexus and is often found in someone who is outwardly self-opinionated and self-assured, but inwardly is hiding poor self-worth and lack of confidence. For many, alcohol gives that confidence but is a crutch rather than reality. Facing the truth usually involves removal of the crutch but can only occur when the individual is ready to build their inner confidence.

Comfort eating can also lead to fat over the solar plexus especially in women. When they feel depressed, tense or unloved, they eat. Chocolates are the common comforter but sugar of any type will do. Others eat starchy foods, bread, pastries, etc. but the end result is the same.

Instead of enhancing self-worth the individual then feels guilty and is depressed by their increase in weight.

Comfort eating is especially common in those who do not wish to speak out for fear it causes an upset. Feed the mouth and stop it speaking. The path to breaking this pattern consists of:

a) Recognising there is a problem and the situations which are more likely to lead to comfort eating.

b) Deciding to change and choosing to talk rather than bottling the emotions.

c) Replacing the activity of eating with another activity involving the hands.

If you must eat, choose something which is least fattening.

It is a common problem especially amongst women who feel things more acutely than men but are not always able to express themselves clearly and objectively. Self-assertion classes have been a great help in this area.

Some Diseases Related to the Solar Plexus

1) Diabetes
There are two types of diabetic patients: those who require insulin, where the disease may be related to an auto-immune problem (making antibodies against self), and those whose cells are no longer sensitive to their own insulin and therefore glucose cannot pass across the cell membrane.

The latter condition is commonly found in the elderly who have had a high sugar intake throughout their life often due to comfort eating. The body simply becomes immune to the sugar.

In both groups there is a tendency towards suppression of emotions and a non-complaining attitude which is seen in their general compliance to a strict diet and medical routines. However, this can lead to emotional manipulation especially around those who are close.

There is also often poor self esteem which is expressed in either strong views and dogmatism to which everybody else has to agree or lack of any valid opinion. Another aspect is their difficulty in forming secure relationships leading to dependency on the parental home which may conversely appear as an apparent independence at an early age.

Diabetics need to know how to communicate their feelings in a balanced manner and to recognise their own self-worth.

The auto-immune situation is more complex and will be discussed under the heart chakra.

2) Other Diseases of the Pancreas

The pancreas is the site for the production of not only insulin but also of the digestive enzymes required to break food down into manageable pieces. This digestion takes place in the mouth, stomach and small intestine.

Without sufficient enzymes, we suffer from indigestion and food may pass unchanged from one end to the other producing diarrhoea with pale, fatty stools, nausea, bloating of the abdomen and excessive wind.

Esoterically, this represents someone who is overwhelmed by the experiences which they have ingested and is unable to deal with the situation. They need to learn not to "bite off more than they can chew" as well as realising that, instead of becoming overwhelmed, they should learn to break the experiences into small portions which are more manageable.

An enzyme is a catalyst and therefore remains unaltered whilst creating change within a given situation. All therapists, whatever their training, should be enzymes, ie. performing their task whilst remaining compassionately detached from the experience.

Pancreatitis is a condition where there is inflammation of the pancreas and the enzymes are freely released into the bloodstream and into the surrounding pancreatic tissues, which they start to digest.

This disease often occurs after trauma, whether emotional or physical, although it is also seen where there is a high alcohol intake. Esoterically, it represents suppressed release of emotions, especially fear, often in a highly sensitive individual. Release needs to be encouraged in order to restore the equilibrium.

3) Liver Disease

The liver has many functions. It is the main detoxification centre within the body and manufactures vitamins and proteins for use by the body. It is also the main centre for the assimilation of foods, turning them into energy and storing this for future use.

Unfortunately, on the emotional level it can store not only positive energies but also those which are negative to the body. The greatest of these in terms of the liver, is suppressed anger. Such problems are common throughout the world, even in societies which appear fairly volatile. In these cases, it is common to find that anger is expressed at everything else except the source of the problem, usually due to the fear of causing distress ... the pleaser syndrome.

These stored emotions will create disharmony within the liver, causing tiredness and digestive disorders.

I have seen cases of clinical hepatitis where no causative organism was found but which followed situations of extreme anger and resentment where these were suppressed in order to keep the peace.

When the toxins of anger accumulate then any foods which also have a toxic effect, eg. "junk" foods, alcohol, fats, coffee, tea and sweets, will lead to further disharmony within the energies of the liver.

Those people with such problems, especially those with "hazel" or green eyes, should partake of a simple diet whilst also dealing with their suppressed anger.

4) Gall Stones

The liver manufactures **bile** which is stored in the **gall bladder**. Bile is required to emulsify the fats within the duodenum so that they can be digested and absorbed for use by the body.

The gall bladder acts as the half-way house between the liver and the gut. Esoterically, it also retains this role between the desire to please and the stored resentment, leading to indecision. Ultimately, the anger is stored in the little bag provided, the gall bladder, so that one day, when you really feel angry, you can take the stones out and throw them at someone! Unfortunately, when the gall bladder is removed, by some kind surgeon, you have to start collecting your specimens all over again!

Such people need help not only to recognise their need to please but also their resentment. Through this they can learn to stand back and act only when they can do this purely from their heart and not through guilt or duty. This takes time and the individual needs the reassurance that it is most unlikely they will ever become uncaring … it is not in their nature.

5) Peptic Ulcer

An ulcer is a break in the surface of a lining whether this is in the stomach, the intestine or the skin. There are two types of peptic ulcers, duodenal and gastric. Their particular features are as follows:

A) Duodenal Ulcer

The pain of this ulcer usually occurs 2 to 4 hours after the intake of food. Sometimes this is later, with a common pattern of waking about 2 am and going downstairs for milk and biscuits.

Psychologically, the individual is usually very conscientious and will work hard at any task without complaint. They appear outwardly to be confident and in control; inwardly they worry they may not reach the standards required and that they may not receive approval for their actions.

In the middle of the night, or when they are relaxing in the evening, their anxieties and concerns, which are "gnawing" away in their intestine, start to make their presence felt. The end-result of both this and a gastric ulcer is a perforation.

Such people would be helped by learning to talk about their feelings or at least by writing them down before they go to bed. In this way, such worries can then be assessed objectively and the appropriate action taken rather than allowing things to magnify within the mind.

The question of the need to be needed and to be perfect also has to be looked at and steps taken to realise one's own inner self-worth and the flexibility to be imperfect.

B) Gastric Ulcer
These people are very different. Their pain occurs almost immediately after food. They may have suffered bouts of gastritis in the past brought on by rich foods, alcohol, spices, coffee, smoking and stress.

This last factor is the greatest cause of their problems; for during an adrenaline drive (which occurs as a reaction to stress) the blood supply and the release of digestive enzymes are reduced leading to the relatively unprotected lining of the stomach being easily destroyed by toxic substances.

Psychologically, these are the "worriers" and instead of releasing their anxieties, they store them in the stomach. Part of the reason behind this action is the fear of speaking out, but often the anxiety has become so much part of their make-up that they would not know what to do if they did not worry. They may even wear the title "worrier" with some pride and will search for hours for someone or something to worry about.

They, too, would be helped to release their concerns through speaking or writing but, in many cases, it is more important to provide them with another identity rather than encouraging their thoughts. This block strongly relates to the throat chakra.

6) Hiatus Hernia and Reflux Oesophagitis
These two conditions can appear together or separately. A hiatus hernia occurs when part of the stomach passes through a weakness in the diaphragm and moves into the chest cavity.

This means that the stomach contents are no longer tightly held within their container and food and acid can then move up and down the oesophagus ... reflux oesophagitis.

The reflux can occur where there is added pressure in the abdomen, eg. during pregnancy, with obesity and during the wearing of tight corsets!

Esoterically, the link is between the solar plexus and the throat and reveals difficulty in expressing one's feelings, exacerbated by a worrying nature.

Release of the anxieties, either verbally or from the thoughts, is the answer to the problem (as well as removing the tight corsets and losing weight!).

7) Coeliac's Disease
The effect of this illness leads to stunting of the villi of the small intestine. These villi are normally finger-like projections which increase the surface area for the absorption of the digested food from the intestine.

The commonest cause of the problem is hyper-sensitivity to a component of the gluten protein found in certain grains, including wheat. Removal of the gluten leads to regeneration of the villi.

Esoterically, failure to absorb food relates to failure or resistance to absorb experiences which may have been painful. This leads physically to diarrhoea which is the body's attempt to remove something which is unpleasant.

Unfortunately, by not absorbing the experiences valuable lessons are lost and the same situations may occur time and time again, creating further pain and insecurity.

Apart from Coeliac's disease, there are many people who are spiritually malnourished as they fail to absorb from life those lessons which, although painful, eventually lead to greater freedom and joy.

8) Diseases Within the Spleen
The spleen is part of the main immune system and is involved with the production of antibodies, removing waste material and the destruction of old cells from the blood.

The physical spleen does not relate precisely to the spleen which is described in oriental medicine. The latter sees the spleen as being involved with the transformation of food into energy as well as regulating the flow of blood.

Emotionally, this spleen is related to thoughtfulness and where there is stagnation of thought there will also be stagnation of digestion and blood flow.

Esoterically, there is a spleen centre, related to the physical spleen. This receives "pranic" energy which is the basic life force found within all living things and, in this way, man is connected to his environment.

It could be said that the spleen is the controller of rhythm beneath the diaphragm, whilst the heart controls the flow above.

When there is disharmony in this area, there can be feelings of loneliness or antagonism towards the rest of the world. There can be altered perception as to that which is being offered and lack of trust.

Guidance is needed to see things as they really are and help given to reconnect with the world, allowing the flow of life to become smooth again.

Exercises to Balance the Solar Plexus

1) Write a list of six talents which you are proud to own and then write a C.V. (curriculum vitae) to God stating why He should employ you!

2) Recognise your need to be needed. Accept that you are worthy to receive love by just being you.

3) Choose to own your feelings and not to become overwhelmed by them. Having acknowledged their presence decide whether you wish to stay "angry, moody, jealous, sad, etc.", ie. to identify with your emotions or to see yourself as more than your feelings and to move forward. If you choose to stay as your emotions; what do you hope to gain from this approach?

4) If you decide to change you may need to express the feelings first. This can be achieved through "writing a letter you never send" (even to those who are dead), talking to the indi-

viduals involved, releasing feelings such as anger by hitting a pillow or shouting (the car is a great place for this) or just by taking back your power, accepting the situation and letting go of the feeling. You cannot change others but you can change the way you wish to live.

When you are in a position where you feel overwhelmed by your emotions find a way of altering the immediate atmosphere, ie. go and make coffee, change the music, wash your hands, etc. This defuses the situation but should be followed immediately by a calm but honest expression of your feelings. (Suppression of emotions drains your energy and it is far more difficult to express them at a later date.)

5) Choose to act unconditionally and without guilt or fear of becoming selfish. True unconditional love is mutually beneficial on a soul level.

6) Only give help and advice when requested. Do not look for your needs to be met in those who do not need your help. You will only be disappointed and let down.

7) If you find expressing feelings is difficult, consciously start your conversion with the words "I feel …". Keep a diary, not of the day's events, but of your feelings.

8) If you are sensitive and easily drained by others' energies, imagine a mirror placed between you and allow all their negative energies to be reflected back rather than reaching your solar plexus.

Any energies which do collect in this area can be visualised and seen to pass out of the body, through the feet and into the earth. The earth is the main transformer and will change these negative energies into something more positive.

9) If you are going into a difficult situation or when you feel stressed, close your solar plexus and work purely through the other chakras, keeping the feet firmly planted on the ground. You can protect the chakra by using a crystal, (cleaning it after the event) or the hands and arms which are also useful tools of protection.

Following the event, or when you feel drained, use running water, eg. hand washing, to change the positive ions into negative ones.

10) Ask yourself why you are so sensitive and start to develop a better sense of self-worth. Maybe it is time to say "No" to situations which cause distress. In other cases it may be time to speak your mind, rather than to stay quiet.

11) If you feel dull and uninspired you can use yellow, the colour of the solar plexus, to lift the energies. On the other hand, too much yellow can lead to exhaustion. Then the colours green and blue can be used to re-create peace and healing.

Summary of the Three Lower Chakras

The Base Chakra is the centre which relates to the will of the personality and shall eventually receive the will of the soul (the Father/Spirit).

The Sacral Chakra relates to the creativity of the personality and shall eventually receive the creative energy of the soul (the Mother/Matter).

The Solar Plexus Chakra relates to meeting the desires of the personality and shall eventually receive and meet the desires, and the needs, of the soul (the Son/Soul).

The power of the will, the power of creativity and the power of attraction are the three attributes of the mind belonging to the Source of all Creation. By revealing these attributes within our lives, we are not only expanding our own soul-consciousness but also the consciousness of all life as we know it.

Chapter 10

The Heart Chakra

THE HEART CHAKRA

Position	:	Centre of Chest
Spiritual Aspect	:	Self-Love
Basic Need	:	To Give and Take
		Unconditionally
Related Emotions	:	Joy, Hurt, Bitterness
Endocrine Gland	:	Thymus
Associated Organs	:	Heart, Breasts
Colour	:	Green

Anatomy of the Thymus

In the infant, the thymus gland covers much of the front of the chest. At puberty it has reached its maximum size and then starts to shrink. Until recently it has been said that the thymus gland atrophies in adult life. However, the AIDS epidemic has led to further research showing that indeed there is activity beyond puberty.

Physiology of the Thymus

The thymus gland is involved with the maturation of certain lymphocytes (white blood cells) and with overall activity of lymphoid tissue. Such tissue enables an individual to recognise self or non-self and to deal with the latter appropriately.

The formation of **antibodies** occurs chiefly in the first seven years of life when an individual is challenged by the large amount of new experiences or **antigens**.

Esoterically, the antibody/antigen response leads to the formation of the belief systems which will guide us through our lives, ie. we learn what is good for us and what to avoid.

How one reacts to an antigen when it is next encountered will very much depend on the original presentation and whether the belief system is updated in response to new information from a soul level.

Energy Transformation from the Solar Plexus to the Heart

The heart is the centre for the reception of the love of the soul and, through the soul, links with the love of the Creator. At present, the heart chakra is relatively closed in most of the population and is therefore not fully receiving the total impact of soul love.

However, as the Aquarian Age approaches there will be a massive increase in the energy entering both our hearts and the heart of the universe. To accommodate this change it is important to start to transmute the energies of the solar plexus into those of the heart.

This process is already taking place as is seen by the increase in diseases relating to the heart and the immune system. These occur in relation to the crisis which is brought about by the change and symbolise a degree of resistance.

The main resistance is in relation to the need to disconnect one's desires from conditions and learn to give and receive freely, trusting that one's needs will always be met. This is unconditional love.

There are very few diseases at present associated purely with the heart chakra; most relate to this transmutation.

Spiritual Aspect ... Self-Love

The concept of self-love has in the past been discouraged as it has been seen as being self-centred and failing to consider the needs of others.

"Love thy neighbour as thyself" is often quoted as a reminder to think of others first (Matthew 22 : 39). But it is the "as thyself" which is forgotten by so many.

How can we hope to love others unconditionally if we are

unable to do the same for ourselves. First, we must learn to love our being and this means "warts and all".

This includes all those parts of which we are not proud: nose, our large thighs, our bust, our ears, followed by: our bad temper, our intolerance, our moodiness, our anger.

To try to ignore these parts and to push them into the shadows is not loving or accepting oneself. We may not like what we see but it is the truth and this needs to be faced. The more they are ignored, the more energy is required to keep them quiet. Hating these parts is time-consuming. Loving them releases the hold and in most cases they then fade into insignificance.

Your acceptance does not mean that you need to give them space to develop. You can then choose not to express them just as you can choose to wear certain clothes without the fear that the unworn clothes will jump out and attack you.

So, during this transformation of energies to the heart chakra, we may be faced with situations in which we are not comfortable. Recognising that this is a stage in development of soul consciousness helps us to let go and to pass through the process with far less discomfort.

Without self-love there is a large dependency on others to provide the love which is needed. Just as with the solar plexus, where the need was to be needed, now the need is to be loved.

These two conditions are interlinked and much of that which has been stated concerning the solar plexus will also relate to this transmutation stage.

The Emotions

When the heart is open and free it emits the feeling of joy. When it is closed, and the flow between the solar plexus and heart is disharmonic, then the feelings which are emitted consist of hurt, vulnerability and sometimes bitterness.

These "negative" emotions can be resolved by letting go of expectations, letting go of past events and letting in love. These stages do not occur without some effort but the joy which results is worth the wait.

Hurt occurs when that which has been expected has not

taken place, leading to disappointment and a feeling of rejection. The expectations may have been on a sub-conscious level but they will still influence the outcome.

"I expected you to be faithful to me". This was never discussed but just assumed.

"I expected you to be there for me when I needed you". Again, often an assumption rather than reality.

"I did not expect you to treat me in this way". That is probably true, but then there are the actions of two people to consider in any relationship.

We have all been hurt in some way or other in our lives. It is not comfortable but through it we learn to love ourselves and not to place so many expectations on others. There are those, however, who go back time and time again, repeating the pattern and becoming more and more disillusioned with life.

The hurt can reach so deeply that bitterness starts to appear. I find that this is one of the most destructive emotions, especially when it has been allowed to develop over many years.

It is very difficult to make these people understand that they have some part to play in the creation of their pain. They can only see it from one viewpoint and cannot understand why their needs were not met. They demand revenge and punishment to those who caused the pain. In some cases one can sympathise with their situation, but the event is over and it is time to let go and move forward.

Cases which are extremely difficult to resolve are those when bitterness is part of the grieving process:

"Why did he leave me when I needed him?"

All the bitterness in the world will not reverse the situation and heaven help him when they meet up again on another plane!

In the end, the bitterness can only hurt one person and that is the sender of the emotion. Eventually, even the body takes on a stiff and twisted shape which symbolises the energy of the mind.

To "forgive and forget" is not easy, especially the forgetting. But time heals the memory so that the pain is less acute; time also releases one from the event so that space can be given for new experiences, ie. for-giving.

Forgiveness means to let go … it does not necessarily mean to condone what has happened but to accept that you no longer wish to be part of the experience.

Everybody is on a soul path and, although we may not like what others do, we must learn to love the soul within and set it free.

Forgiveness must also include the self; there is often blame apportioned to the event and although once again you may not wish to condone your behaviour it is time to accept what has been learnt and to move forward.

Hurt is often related to vulnerability.

"I opened my heart to him; I thought I could trust him. He let me down. Now I feel so vulnerable and I do not know if I will ever be able to trust again".

Love is strongly linked with trust. But, in many, there is such an eagerness to find the love which they never received in childhood that they lay themselves open to hurt. No other person can love you as much as you can; no other person fully knows your needs; no other person can be as close.

"He gives me all the material gifts I could desire and yet I am so unhappy. All I want is his closeness and his love".

In an attempt to draw these out of a partner or relative, the individual can open themselves to abuse and poor self-worth. When they are denied, one is left shaken and vulnerable.

The immediate response, like the crab, is to return within the shell and to hide. However, as time passes, one forgets what it is like to be outside and believes that this solitary environment is reality.

Many individuals who have been hurt by the human race turn to the plant and animal kingdoms for their love. Nature is forgiving, faithful and provides unconditional love. They find themselves weeping when watching programmes concerned with suffering especially when it involves animals and children. They are weeping for their own inner child who is vulnerable, often alone and needs love.

They believe that nobody loves them but it is usually the case that the shell, which is keeping pain out, is also keeping love out. With gentle love and encouragement, they need to be persuaded to allow a small part of themselves to be nurtured and, in this way, learn to trust again.

Self-love is to learn to attract towards you those things which are needed and to deny those things which are not needed. By hiding within a shell or opening oneself fully into a situation, we swing between the extremes of all or nothing.

We need to learn discernment which means to use insight to decide that which is good and that which is bad. This is not judgement for we cannot judge the actions of another without this judgement reflecting part of ourselves.

"Judge not, that ye be not judged" (Matthew 7 : 1).

No discernment can lead to a total lack of opinion and lack of boundaries. The energy of the heart chakra is to learn balance. We should love all souls equally as brothers, but we do not always have to like the personality!

Fear of becoming vulnerable leads to an individual choosing a career where there is little personal involvement. Such people may be wonderful listeners, always hearing about the problems of others, but rarely revealing their own inner feelings. When asked personal questions they answer with a question, turning the conversation away from themselves.

There is a great fear of being judged and through this judgement to be rejected and unloved. And yet if you ask them if they reject their friends when things go wrong, they answer "Oh no, I always forgive them and love them more".

It is hard for them to see that the same principles would probably apply in their case if only they would allow people to come close.

Such people may have many acquaintances but few true friends; people with whom they can safely open their hearts. They would rather be in the company of strangers than with friends. The latter brings the risk of expectations and of possible failure.

All that one can offer as an outsider, is unconditional love which shows that whichever way they choose to turn, love and support is always at hand.

The ability to give unconditionally is often easier than to receive. The latter needs true self-love and to realise that when you are receiving, you are receiving not only for yourself, but for your Creator.

Some people, on being given a present, will almost ignore this item in their anxiety to find something to repay the debt. They also find it difficult to receive compliments and will immediately return it, often in a more expansive manner.

They do not realise that to deny the gift is to deny the giver.

Unconditional love is not giving in. A mother bird will push her young out of the nest in the name of love, even though their wings are not fully formed. Sometimes one needs to be cruel, to be kind.

When there are issues around love, it is best to find a quiet spot and, whilst sitting, reach to your higher self and ask for a solution which will be best for all concerned.

In this way, the answer should be objective and create movement for all along their paths. It does not mean that there may not be pain, but holding on to the solution gives you strength to carry the project through to the end.

Courage is the essence of the heart (coeur ... the heart). We all need courage at certain times and can be supported by the en-couragement of others along our path. When there is no encouragement, then it feels there is no love and one expresses discouragement. Honest encouragement is one of the greatest gifts we can give to another person.

In the desire to be loved we can often take on more responsibility than we can handle. The issue of responsibility comes under the Third Eye chakra but when we are blinded by our needs this centre loses control.

Responsibility for others, which starts as a good cause, can soon become like an albatross around the neck, weighing one down and sapping the energy. As with the pleaser, resentment can build, but more often there is a feeling of despair and a fear that there will be no solution to the problem.

In the end, the only way out for many is through illness as will be discussed under the heading of diseases of the heart. Self-love means self-preservation and without this we cannot offer help to anyone else.

Body Language

We have all seen children who have been rebuked standing in a corner with their hands across their chest. They are nursing their painful heart and this habit is carried into adult life whenever there is a need for comfort.

We also talk about being touched by someone's kindness and this sense is strongly connected with the heart. There are many people nowadays who are rarely touched and if they are it is only in a sexual manner. Touch has become one of the most important features of complementary therapies involving cancer and AIDS, patients often seen as "untouchable".

Hopefully, as the field of holistic medicine widens, we will start to see massage and other touch therapies as part of every patient's care.

Some Diseases Related to the Heart Chakra

1) Heart Disease

The heart is the organ of rhythm. It projects the blood, plus all that it carries, around the body, reaching every single cell. Its impulse has two phases: systole or contraction of the ventricles, and diastole or relaxation.

A complete cycle lasts for 0.8 secs with each phase taking approximately 0.4 secs, ie. half the time is spent in activity and half in relaxation.

Is this true of your life? Do you spend 12 hours a day working and 12 hours relaxing? If not, the heart is under pressure.

The heart muscle receives its nourishment during diastole and, if this phase is deficient, then the oxygen supply to the tissues is also deficient, which could lead to angina and possibly a heart attack (myocardial infarct or coronary thrombosis).

This deficiency is exacerbated by blockage of the coronary arteries with atheroma (fatty deposits) and thrombosis (blood clots). These are commonly caused by high cholesterol levels (80% of which is made during stress) and sluggish blood flow (due to poor exercise).

These factors would be reduced if true relaxation were carried out. By this I mean relaxation of the mind, the body and the spirit. Relaxation cannot occur if time is set against distance, for immediately the brain is active in order to achieve the goal. Similarly, it is also no use forcing the mind to relax, for again the brain will rebel.

Stress management courses are now widely available and will hopefully not only teach the participants to deal with stress but to learn how to live a fuller life.

Esoterically, hardening of the arteries (artherosclerosis) signifies the inflexibility of the situation. In many cases, the individual has taken on too much responsibility and does not know how to stop.

They are walking into a cul-de-sac and there appears to be no turning back. Sometimes, a heart attack is the only way out.

Others have a hardened attitude, often due to lack of love and closeness in their childhood. This symbolically leads to lack of nurturing for their heart muscle, eventually leading to the symptoms.

There is much evidence to show that those who suffer from a heart attack feel isolated prior to the attack, and those who do well following the attack are those who have a loving partner at home.

Love, whether from another or more importantly from self, is very important to the function of the heart.

2) Diseases of the Immune System

There has been a large increase in these diseases in the last 10 years, which relates to the shift in energies. The allergies and hyper-sensitivities are due to an over-sensitive immune system whilst the cancers, AIDS and M.E. are due to a deficiency or under-active immune system. The immune system, as stated above, is the guard at the front door of the body. It recognises friend or foe, admitting the former and rejecting the latter. Disharmony within this guard leads to the following diseases:

A) Allergies and Hyper-Sensitivity

40% of the British public now suffers from some allergy. Allergy is said to be a disease which runs in families, whereas hyper-sensitivity occurs out of the blue.

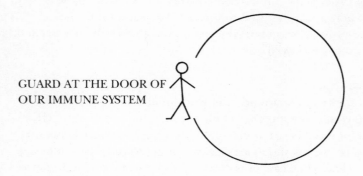

GUARD AT THE DOOR OF
OUR IMMUNE SYSTEM

Both diseases are caused by an over-active immune system, leading to various symptoms such as hay fever, asthma, diarrhoea, eczema and urticaria.

Esoterically, the little guard is over-sensitive and is reacting as if everything is frightening. This is symbolic of the over-sensitivity discussed in the section on the solar plexus. It is as though the world is a frightening place and that only by keeping very alert can one avoid being harmed. Such stress increases the reactions, leading to further problems.

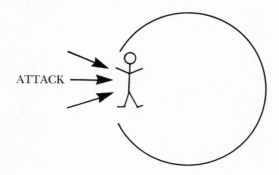

ATTACK

I believe that we are going to see more of these problems as man's sensitivity heightens to reach the incoming energies of the soul.

Through visualisation, the excessive energy within the solar plexus can be diffused into the heart or down into the ground where it can be used to the benefit of the individual. In this way, the fear will be reduced and the guard will once again be able to discern friend from foe.

B) Cancer

Cancer can be found in practically any organ. Therefore, esoterically, the links are made through the appropriate chakra. However, there is usually an underlying imbalance between the solar plexus and heart chakra leading to cellular changes.

The name cancer is derived from the crab, denoting movement in any direction. Cancer has the capacity to spread anywhere in the body using the blood and lymph systems.

On a cellular level, normal cells grow and mature, following the rules of the body by not over-stepping their boundaries and by maintaining the same size and shape as their neighbours. Cancer cells do not mature and therefore do not follow the rules. They may have more than one nucleus, take on a strange shape and certainly break the boundaries.

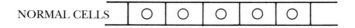

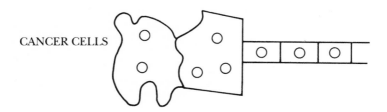

It is the task of our little guard to stop these runaway cells; but, for some reason, he does not notice their misbehaviour. Once the cells have left their "primary" site of development they move on to other organs; there they succeed in persuading normal cells to turn over their DNA production to the production of more cancer cells. In this way "secondaries" are produced.

Psychospiritually this reveals certain issues about the personality. One image is that the guard has left his post in order to help other people. This is indeed the case for many cancer patients who are always working to help others but, in doing so, leave their own defences weak.

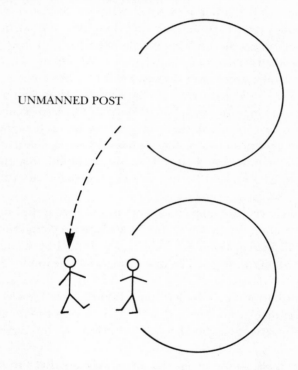

UNMANNED POST

It is a case of "while the cat is away, the mice will play" and reminds one that love must start at home.

An Analogy

A group of people work on a production line removing "bad peas" from the line before the "good peas" pass into a common pot.

One person spends so much time helping others that she fails to notice the bad peas which enter the pot from her own production line.

By not taking care of her own line, she jeopardizes the whole process.

The American psychologist Lawrence Le Shan wrote in his book "You can Fight for Your Life" that many cancer patients were "not singing their own song". They were living their life through others and denying their own needs.

This brings up another point which is the fact that when you are not fully present within your body, then there is no strong regulating force to decide what is right and what is wrong.

As described earlier, those who have a good prognosis from cancer are the fighters and the deniers. They take control of their lives. Those who do badly are those who feel hopeless and those who exhibit stoic acceptance. As with all diseases, cancer does not necessarily mean that changes must occur, for sometimes the very presence of the disease will bring about the changes which the soul desires. However, it should be a time of reflection to check whether there are areas of one's life which are being ignored.

For cancer certainly appears in organs related to unfinished business and especially where there are suppressed emotions. It can be likened to a child who is being ignored. The less attention, the louder it shouts. The more you shout, the louder the noise.

The disharmonic cells, like the children, need to have their presence acknowledged and harmony restored, not through anger or guilt, but through loving but structured guidance.

Cancer is also known to appear up to two years after the loss of an identity linked with the death of a partner, loss of a job, the children leaving home, etc. This relates back to the solar plexus/heart interaction where identity and love are closely linked. Loss of the former appears to lead to loss of the latter.

Let us hope that through the development of self-worth and self-love, there will be a reduction in the incidence of cancer in society.

Cancer of the Breast

The breast is the organ of nurturing. In cancer of the breast, it is this issue which is out of balance.

In my own experience, I have found that those with left-sided breast cancer often feel unsupported and unloved by the men in their life, whether it is a husband or father. Those with right-sided breast cancer feel hurt through the actions of a woman, which can be a mother or daughter.

Both need to recognise their own nurturing abilities and to release the hurt which they are holding within their breast.

C) AIDS

The AIDS virus attacks the ability of the thymus gland to make T-helper cells (CD4), which are required in almost every immune response. Those people who manifest the disease are therefore presented with a multitude of infections and tumours, which in normal circumstances would be eradicated by our little guard.

Psychologically, it has been noted that many of the sufferers are minority groups and therefore often seen as "victims" of society, eg. the homosexuals, drug addicts and even the haemophiliacs.

As individuals, there is often a history of poor encouragement and nurturing when young, leading to poor self-worth in adult life. Their little guard becomes despondent.

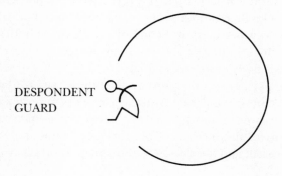

DESPONDENT
GUARD

It has been clearly shown that unconditional love and the encouragement of self-love help in the remission of symptoms. This is especially the case with the children who have been lucky enough to find a home where they can receive such love. Nowadays, it is the AIDS wards which are most commonly visited by the complementary therapists. It is ironic to think that a disaster such as AIDS should be a major key to the introduction of complementary medicine into the hospitals.

AIDS is a disease of victims; those sections of society which are unloved. Where in your body is your "AIDS"? Look inside and discover those areas which are waiting to be nurtured and lavish them with love.

D) Auto-Immune Diseases

This group of illnesses includes rheumatoid arthritis, systemic lupus erythematosus (SLE), scleroderma, systemic sclerosis, polymyalgia rheumatica, some types of thyroid disease, some forms of diabetes, pernicious anaemia and vitiligo. More are being added to the list every month.

The common bond in all cases is that an antibody has been made against the individual's own tissues. For example, in rheumatoid arthritis the antibody is against the joint lining and other lining tissues. In SLE, the antibody is against the DNA of the cells.

These are fairly powerful methods of destroying oneself and psychologically there is often a strong essence of the "martyr syndrome" within these people. It is very difficult to persuade them to change their attitudes away from their low self-worth.

They usually work hard on behalf of others, denying their own needs. But eventually these needs do emerge, not clearly, but often in a fairly desperate manner.

It is so important as a therapist to meet these patients half way. This encourages movement on the part of the sufferer and prevents the carer becoming entwined in a process which can be destructive to all concerned. There is a large element of the "pleaser" present and this should be discouraged and replaced with self-love.

Many do choose to change their attitudes although it is a

struggle as it means changing the habits of a lifetime. They need constant reassurance and encouragement but must not be carried if at all possible.

E) Myalgia Encephalomyelitis (M.E.)

This disease, also known as **chronic fatigue syndrome and post-viral syndrome**, is an illness which is gaining momentum within the Western societies.

In affects the muscles and the brain, leading to extreme exhaustion, muscle weakness and muscle pains. There are many other symptoms, some of which are involved with an overgrowth of the yeast, candida.

There are various phases of the disease and its underlying cause is not entirely clear. It can occur at any age, in both sexes and affects all walks of life. Some patients are bed-bound by their weakness and extreme lethargy, others are mobile but experience severe pains and headaches. It is possible that we will find that there are different types of illness under the common heading.

Psychospiritually, the pattern which I have observed is that this disease seems to affect those who are not walking on their own path. They are often pleasers, acting in accordance with the wishes of others. They are going in one direction miles away from their planned path. This disorientation leads to the tiredness and weakness as there is no real soul energy entering their body.

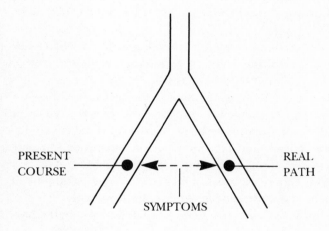

PRESENT COURSE — REAL PATH — SYMPTOMS

The illness allows them time to take stock of the situation and to change direction if required. In many cases friends disappear, showing the true level of love which was available. I have found that until the patient accepts that they are ill, the illness steadily gets worse. The day they admit that things must change, the illness starts to recede. This does not, however, happen overnight and patience is one of the words which M.E. sufferers are always hearing in connection with their recovery.

To know what is right for you, after years of doing what was right for everybody else, takes time and deep thought but slowly the path reappears, as does health. Perhaps the only lesson that these people were meant to learn whilst on this earth was self-love. If they achieve this, then they are truly rich.

Exercises to Balance the Solar Plexus/Heart Interaction

1) Start to love yourself by loving your physical body, your sacred temple; it is the only one you will be given on this journey. If you cannot love all the lumps and bumps, start with a small section such as your little finger. Use pleasant smelling oils and rub these into your body, affirming that you love it.

2) Make a contract to allow yourself one indulgence during the day/week/month (make the goal achievable), eg. to have a long soak in the bath; to read a good novel; to sit down to eat; to walk at lunchtime; to have a holiday this year.

3) Affirm your desire for true love: "I am loved, I am lovable, I am love".

4) Use the colour green to harmonise the heart. This can be achieved by wearing green or by walking in nature. Nature works in cycles and reveals the rhythm of life.

5) You may choose to use pink as the heart chakra colour and this can be achieved through rose quartz crystals or through clothes or house decor. Whenever there is conflict, visualise yourself and the other person surrounded in pink blankets symbolising unconditional love.

6) Where there are areas of hurt in your body, send pink or gold light to remove the pain and renew the energy.

7) Choose to forgive someone who has hurt you in the past.

You may wish to write a letter you never send or to visualise the person sitting opposite and tell them how you feel. Remember also to meet them at the place of their higher self and send them love as a soul on their future path.

8) As with the solar plexus, learn to say "No". When asked a favour, stall for time by saying that you must think about it or consult your diary before committing yourself.

Then, in the space which has been developed, ask your higher self whether you are doing this favour from your heart or from your desire to please. If the latter is true, decline the offer or choose to change your desire. This same procedure can be used whenever there is a tendency to say "Yes" without forethought.

Chapter 11

The Throat Chakra

THE THROAT CHAKRA

Position : Throat
Spiritual Aspect : Self-Expression
Basic Need : Ability to Accept Change
Related Emotions : Frustration, Freedom
Endocrine Gland : Thyroid Gland
Associated Organs : Lung, Throat, Intestines
Colour : Blue

Anatomy of the Thyroid Gland
The thyroid gland is situated over the lower, anterior portion of the neck, lying over the trachea.

Physiology of the Thyroid Gland
This gland produces thyroxine (T4) and other related hormones which are involved in generating activity within the cells, promoting growth and repair. It is particularly active around periods of change such as puberty and the menopause and disfunction is often seen at these times.

Spiritual Aspect ... Self-Expression

My Will Versus Thy Will
The evolvement of the animal kingdom led to man who functions not only through the astral body but also with the aid of an ever-developing mental body. This body provides logical and analytical thought and, through these mechanisms, protects the individual from the effects of an over-developed astral body.

An impulse from the soul, which is an expression of the higher Self, enters the chakra system through the crown centre and the right cerebral hemisphere. From here, it passes down to the throat chakra where it is converted into a thought-form. This is then taken up by the astral body and is expressed through the heart or solar plexus centres, depending on whether the impulse is now satisfying the needs of the soul or of the personality.

This transfer of control often takes place in the throat chakra where the personality of man has learnt to use the power of the mental body to its own advantage. Therefore, when the impulse from the soul is presented at this centre, it may be challenged if it does not conform to the plans and belief systems of the personality.

Such a challenge means that the impulse may be blocked at the throat and passed back through the crown via the left cerebral hemisphere. This action can stunt soul growth and lead to conflict between the will of the personality and the will of the soul, which can in time manifest as physical disease in the area of the throat chakra.

I find that this chakra is one which is commonly out of balance as man learns to use his mental body for the creative expression not only of the desires of the personality but also those of the soul.

The Breath of Life

The impulse of the soul is received as **inspiration**. It heralds the birth of the manifestation of a new idea. Symbolically, it is represented in the physical body by the in-breath (inhalation) which is also called inspiration.

Through the creation of the thoughtform, this impulse is structured and can now be expressed in words or actions. The reaction to its release forms the basis for the creation of a new impulse, ie. the completion or death of one impulse (expiration) leads to the birth of another (inspiration). Between the birth and the death is a momentary pause which signifies the time taken to assimilate the information received from one impulse before creating another.

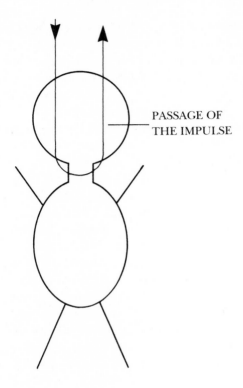

PASSAGE OF
THE IMPULSE

BLOCKED THROAT CHAKRA

In physical terms, the out-breath (exhalation), or expiration, represents the expression of the thoughtform. It is followed by a pause while a small sensor in the neck, called the carotid body, assesses the level of the gases in the blood stream. Rising carbon dioxide and falling oxygen levels act as the trigger to stimulate the start of another cycle through inspiration.

Esoteric studies suggest that there is a link between the carotid body, the pituitary and pineal glands which together represent the regulation of the expression, reception and creation of the impulse.

We breathe eighteen times per minute. Each cycle represents a birth and a death, with a wealth of experience in between.

Sound as a Form of Expression

The two vocal cords are attached to part of the larynx which comes under the influence of the throat chakra. We speak by using the breath of exhalation and passing it between the cords which have been brought closer together by the use of laryngeal muscles.

The ears are organs of balance and hearing. For children, hearing is vitally important in the development of speech. A deaf child will have difficulty with pronunciation and will speak in a monotonous tone.

The ears allow us to hear our own speech and to check, on a deeper level, if that which we express is true to the original impulse. There is a strong connection between tinnitus and the failure to hear and express the true impulse (see later).

Related Emotions

I always know if someone has problems with their throat chakra after a short conversation. It is the chakra of **excuses**.

They are the "yes, but ..." people. Before you are half way through suggesting a solution to their problem, they are impatient to answer you with "yes, but the buses don't run on a Sunday" or "yes, but the cat needs feeding" or "yes, but it might snow in the middle of June".

It is fascinating to listen to them; never before has there been such a selection of excuses:

"I'm too busy helping others" ... makes them believe that they are very important and self-sacrificing.

"I'm too tired" ... caused by the boredom and continual effort of making excuses.

"It's too difficult".

"I won't be able ...".

"I can't" ... before they even try.

Then there are the excuses which relate to the future:

"When the children leave home, then I'll ...".

"When my husband retires, then I'll ...".

"When I win money, then I'll ...".

"When I run out of excuses, then I'll ...".

In all these cases, the analytical processes of the mental body are being used to manipulate the situation to the advantage of the personality. These people are logical in their thinking and will usually start their sentences with: "I think …".

It is no use trying to argue with them for they will have a string of answers to defeat your questions. The best thing to do is to agree with them and wait until they are ready to change. They can be very stubborn and defensive for, like those with base and the solar plexus problems, they need to be in control.

The excuses are used as a means of preventing inner self-expression caused by a variety of underlying fears:

"If I say what I think, will people still like me?"

"If I speak my mind, will I be understood?"

"If I let people know who I really am, will I be accepted?"

"If I say what I want, will I be seen as being selfish?"

"If I say what I feel, will I hurt others?"

All these comments are related to other chakras where the issues are around self-worth, self-love, self-respect, etc. But in the end, it is the throat chakra which has control over self-expression as it encompasses one of the most important means of communication.

Here we see the tie between the sacral and throat chakras. Both relate to communication and expression through a common bond. In the sacral chakra the bond is between two people or the male and female aspects of ourselves. In the throat chakra the bond is between the personality and the soul.

Many people find it difficult to shift the energies from the sacral to the throat; from "myself as part of a relationship", to "myself as part of the soul energy". This is particularly common in menopausal women who have created their children but do not know how to create themselves.

The reverse occurs in those who have problems with sexual identity and forming heterosexual relationships. Here, the energy of the sacral chakra is transferred into the throat leading to a high level of creative output, eg. through music, art, poetry, dancing, hair dressing. But one chakra cannot be developed to the exclusion of another; eventually the balance must be redressed.

Suppression of expression leading to weeping and moodiness

Many women find that instead of becoming angry, they cry, which leads to further frustration as their ability to communicate coherently disappears. They may then be seen as "an emotional woman" rather than someone who can take part in a serious discussion. This may be a throw back to childhood when the woman's point of view was always ignored or seen as being far too emotional.

Weeping is often used by children who cry rather than say what is on their mind. They feel that they would not be understood or heard and this is particularly common where the parents communicate through shouting.

Other children and adults who feel unable to express themselves become moody and turn inwards. It is commonly not clear in their own minds what they are actually trying to say and they may sense that the environment is hostile to any new thoughts or discussions which may involve feelings.

It is so important in any relationship to allow each to express themselves fully, without the partner becoming victim to that which is expressed. This does not mean that they cannot reply, but they should speak from an objective position rather than that of the victim.

Everybody needs to be heard, even children whose speech may be limited and cover "irrelevant" facts. Space should be made in the day so that members of a family, or those in a work place, can talk not only about facts but also feelings.

Change

One of the greatest fears held in the three dominant chakras (base, solar plexus and throat) is the fear of change. Change can lead to insecurity, vulnerability and confusion and for people who like to be in control, these are states which are not welcomed.

Analytical thought, and its expression in the form of speech, can be cleverly used to prevent any change taking place.

There are two main groups of people in this category: those

who are "too busy" to change and those who are "too lazy" to change. Both are avoiding the issue.

Those who are "too busy" will rush into the room, sit on the edge of the chair, speak very quickly as they tell you how much they do in a day and leave little space for your questions. When you do manage to get a word in edgeways about their own self-development, they change the subject or tell you that they must be going.

They may say that they are always changing, and indeed there will be frequent changes within the design of their house, the style of their hair, the location of their home, the layout of their garden and their choice of job. But in the end there may be no movement at all for they are keeping so busy externally that they are avoiding the issues of inner change and expression of the Self.

There is a similar avoidance found in those who are "too lazy or inactive to move". They will slump in the chair, sigh deeply and ask what can you do to make them better. When asked what they are doing, they sigh again and say that they have no energy to move.

Every suggestion that you make is defeated and you start to see why they are so tired. They are expending all their energy in maintaining the facade of laziness.

Both have a fear of facing up to reality:

"Where am I going? I know I'm off my path and that I'm not fulfilled and yet I am scared of making the move towards change".

It may appear that others are resisting our changes which leads to a sense of frustration; this is one of the commonest feelings that I hear being expressed by my patients, but in the end, the frustration is really with our own sense of inadequacy and represents much deeper fears:

"What if my husband won't let me go out to work?" He has never been asked but there is a fear of stepping outside boundaries which are acceptable.

"Nobody in my office supports my move". You are unlikely to receive support from those who may also be stuck.

"What if I fail?" And what if you don't? Fear of failure relates to the base and the need to be perfect. If you never try, you never fail; but you will also lack fulfilment. Choose to give yourself praise for doing the best that you can and let this be the success that you seek.

"I don't think I will make the grade".

Don't set yourself up to fail. Prepare the ground rather than allowing fate to take over. Fate is governed by the power of attraction and therefore can come from the level of the soul or from the level of the personality.

"My family do not understand my desire for change".

That may be true, but does it matter? What matters is that you, on some level, understand the need for self-expression.

"I don't want to hurt others by my selfishness".

As seen in the solar plexus, if we try to please others we end up resenting their needs. Who knows? Having the courage to change may give others the strength to do the same.

Change is not easy, but it is inevitable. It is a part of soul growth and without it we will stagnate. Resisting change can lead to a crisis in our lives which may manifest as disease. This can then be used as the means by which change will take place.

The first step from a position of safety results in a momentary insecurity when there is free flow and the opportunity to go in any direction.

An analogy
When we change gear in a car we always pass through the central point of neutrality. In this position the car is free wheeling and the gears no longer control its actions.

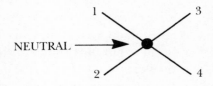

The time of free-wheeling is a time to test belief in one's own soul guidance.

An analogy
Having jumped out of the aeroplane there is a period of free fall when one has to trust that when the cord is pulled the parachute will open.

During this period of neutrality, which may be seen as loss of control, you may decide to jump back to the starting point or to move forward.

Many people do return to the original position only to find that things have not altered and that the same pressures to move are still present. Therefore they jump again, this time passing through the neutral point into safety.

I have seen this pattern in attempts to leave jobs, partners and the family home. There is an initial break, which may be caused by anger or fear, followed by a short return and then a much stronger resolve to leave.

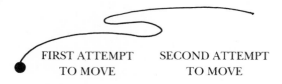

FIRST ATTEMPT   SECOND ATTEMPT
   TO MOVE   TO MOVE

Change is a time of letting go of the old and accepting the new. It is seen symbolically in the snake when it sheds its skin at the beginning of a new cycle of life.

The phase of neutrality, and possible vulnerability, may require a period of hibernation or finding a place of quiet retreat. Here, it is safe to go within and to find the strength and wisdom required for the next move.

This is symbolised by the onset of winter which is a time of reflection and planning before the new birth in the Spring. It is also seen in the caterpillar when it becomes encased in the chrysalis which protects it during the period of metamorphosis, before it emerges as a butterfly.

In a similar way, when a crab wants to expand in size it needs to remove its hard shell so that the inner body can grow. To do this it finds a deep, dark recess where it can be safe, and removes the shell. At this stage it is extremely vulnerable and is hopefully well hidden from view. Slowly, the body increases in size, its thin outer covering starts to harden and take on the shape of the new shell.

Man's strength lies within. Any outer shell will always show weaknesses and can easily be destroyed. Much of our change is related to replacing the outer shell with that supplied by our own inner being.

During times of change it is important to be surrounded by friends and family who love you for "just being you" as well as remembering to nurture the inner child who may be frightened. This means plenty of good food, fresh air, friends, treats and rest periods.

As the "butterfly" emerges, there may be a period of "spring cleaning" when that which is no longer required is released to make way for the new. Unless we make space, by clearing out cupboards which are full of old memories and emotions, there will never be room for new experiences.

Change is often accompanied by a period of grief which follows any loss whether it is that of a relative, partner, job or identity. Even the fact that you missed the train shows a short period of grief. It is the method by which we accept and acknowledge the loss, moving through a variety of emotions which include:

a) **Numbness** where every action is automatic
b) **Guilt and blame** often using phrases such as "if only …"
c) **Anger** at others such as the medical staff or even at the relative who died
d) **Confusion and disorientation** as the actual loss starts to be felt
e) **Acceptance** with the realisation that life must go on

It is easy to become blocked in one phase of the grief period especially when we grieve for our loss rather than the loss of the life of the individual who died. This needs gentle understanding whilst encouraging the need to move forward.

Blocks can appear as disharmony within the physical body. Thus we see unshed tears appearing as a chronic post nasal drip; hurt and guilt often accompanying cancer; anger represented by liver and gall bladder problems; and confusion, related to the third eye manifesting as headaches and visual disturbances.

Only when there is acceptance of the situation and the decision to release the old emotions, will these symptoms disappear.

Inner change is often accompanied by outer changes. These include new clothes, new hairstyles, new decor, new friends, new jobs and new food habits. They all help to solidify the inner change into reality and should be encouraged.

Sometimes old habits, such as alcohol intake, can no longer be tolerated by the new vibration of the inner bodies. This needs to be accepted, for things can never be the same again. Each second brings new experiences, ones which we have never before faced.

Have the courage to change when the soul impulse arrives.

Body Language

The language of the throat can often be revealed through speech. "Something is stuck in my throat", when there is fear of speaking out; "there is a lump in my throat", which often relates to unspoken grief; or there may be a continual need to clear the throat as if about to speak but nothing happens.

Sometimes I see the throat being rubbed during a conversation which represents something which is painful and difficult to express. At other times, a hand is placed over the mouth in an attempt to stop or muffle words coming out which may not be accepted.

People who are inclined to blush may find that their redness stops as it reaches the neck; this signifies a desire to speak, but fear of creating disharmony with those concerned.

I have also noticed that those who do not want to accept new ideas, or who are resistant to change, will wear tight clothing at their necks or surround this area with scarves and high collars.

The opposite is seen in someone who feels trapped and needs to change but cannot see the way to freedom. This is especially common at the time of the menopause, when the suppressed energy of change results in hot flushes, aching muscles, irritability and depression.

These people need loose clothes especially at their neck ... like the snake they cannot bear to be trapped.

The movement of the mouth also shows interesting patterns. For instance, is the mouth used symmetrically during speech? Some people speak out of only one side of the mouth. This shows a fear or anxiety in using the other side and, when it is the right side which is suppressed, it represents difficulties in being assertive. When there is left-sided suppression, there may be fears in expressing one's sensitivities.

The muscles of the jaw and those around the temporo-mandibular joint are sites where anger is commonly held. Tension in these regions can lead to pain in the face, the teeth, the ears and the neck. The mouth has something to say but is being prevented by the inner fear of losing control. A good shout can do a power of good.

Others "bite their tongue" both physically and metaphorically and need to learn to let go. Grinding of the teeth at night suggests inner frustrations which are being stored in the subconscious during the day, only emerging at rest. Keeping a journal or writing down any thoughts before going to bed, certainly helps to relieve tensions and aids sleep and recuperation.

The ears also come under the control of the throat chakra and someone who places their hands over their ears when you are talking says much about their unwillingness to hear what is being said.

Some Diseases Related to the Throat Chakra

1) Hypothyroidism (Myxoedema)
Here there is underactivity of the thyroid gland with a reduction in the levels of thyroxine and other hormones leading to

a slowing down of the metabolic rate. The signs of the disease include weight gain, drying of the hair and skin, constipation, hair loss, intolerance of the cold and depression.

Sub-clinical hypothyroidism is very common (that which does not present as a clinical disease). We all have times when we slump or feel that we cannot move. We put on weight, we are tired and we become a "blob". Blood thyroxine levels are usually normal, but the level of energy through the throat chakra is low. This is commonly a sign of the need to change but where there is some resistance represented as frustration.

The creative urge can be re-ignited by participating in activities such as pottery, art, dancing, singing, writing poetry, etc., which connect the right side of the brain, which receives the soul's impulses, to the units of expression: the hands, the feet and the mouth, hopefully by-passing the logical thought of the left brain.

Thyrotoxicosis
In this disease there is an overactivity of the thyroid gland with weight loss, sweating, tremor, anxiety and palpitations. Here excessive energy is expanded on non-creative activities.

Therapy is required not only to reduce this metabolic rate physically but also to help the individual to focus their energy more creatively using the activities described above.

As with the under-active thyroid, many people show signs of an over-active thyroid without abnormal blood levels. These are times when they are extremely busy trying to do many things at once and perhaps trying to avoid the deeper issues of their own self creativity.

Supporting someone while they stop and look within is the gift that can be offered at this time.

3) Asthma
Asthma is the constriction of the bronchial airways by tight muscles or excess mucus, leading to problems mainly in expiration. These people may have other allergic diseases and are commonly very sensitive emotionally to the en-

vironment, tuning into and reacting to the moods of others.

They believe that there is no room to express their thoughts and feelings and that if they were expressed they may not be accepted.

It is not uncommon to hear that asthma starts in a child during a time of disharmony within the home:

"My first asthma attack happened when I was sitting on my parents' bed and they were arguing".

"My asthma is always worse when I feel that I am not understood".

I have also seen asthma occur in babies where their mother has been anxious during the pregnancy and this has been conveyed to the foetus who, although sensitive to the needs of the mother, is helpless to act.

It is important to teach these children how to protect themselves, especially the area of the solar plexus, from the emotional release of others. They also need to be taught how to express their own feelings freely without the fear of inciting anger and anxiety in those who listen. How the listeners react is their own problem and parents of asthmatic children should be encouraged to offer support to any form of creative expression.

Asthma may also start in adult life after an event where grief is suppressed. Talking, writing and deep breathing are essential for these people.

Most asthmatics, and many anxious people, breathe only in the top of their lungs, with the lower portion held static. The diaphragm, the large muscle at the base of the chest cavity, should move down during inspiration which aids breathing as well as massaging the organs of the abdomen.

Sitting centrally under this muscle is the solar plexus containing many emotions. Splinting the diaphragm and restricting its movement therefore prevents it touching this centre and inadvertently releasing the emotions.

Deep diaphragmatic breathing not only helps to relax the person with asthma, but also aids the expression of the suppressed emotions. This can lead to remission of symptoms for a long period of time.

4) Bronchitis and Emphysema

Bronchitis is inflammation of the bronchii (the breathing tubes) leading to a chronic cough and the production of sputum. It commonly occurs in those who smoke or who are passive smokers. Smoking is a form of suppression of speech and acts like a "dummy" when there is a desire to express oneself but anxiety prevents the action.

I personally have nothing against smoking, but I always ask my patients the reason why they need to smoke. If it is purely social, then they would probably smoke up to 5 cigarettes per day. More than five must be a crutch. However, it is important not to remove one crutch without replacing it with inner strength otherwise a new crutch will appear, eg. over-eating, alcohol or drugs.

Psychospiritually, bronchitis represents a resistance not of expression, but rather of inspiration. They do not want to accept the impulses from their own soul.

Emphysema is the irreversible stage of bronchitis and other serious lung disorders. Pathologically, it is represented by dilated airways, trapped air and collapse of certain areas of the lung. All the inspiration is trapped and this is often seen in the despair of suffering combined with a stubbornness to change patterns of a lifetime.

Most lung disease is related to change and the grief and anxiety that this entails.

5) Sore Throats

When anything is red and inflamed there is a correlation between the physical state and unexpressed anger. In the throat area this is particularly significant as things which should be said are repressed for fear of the reaction. This is even more significant when there is an associated loss of voice.

Learning to speak out, clearly and objectively is the answer to the problem.

6) Tonsillitis

The tonsils, like the adenoids, are part of the immune system. In childhood they are developed to allow the individual to recognise what is usefully acceptable and what to reject.

This process should be complete by the age of nine after which both groups of tissue should become smaller and less functional.

Continuous inflammation of the tonsils represents a continual fear of accepting new experiences or their own creativity. Here the best forms of release of the emotions may be through singing or writing.

7) Hearing Problems
The causes of such diseases are many. These include congenital abnormalities, middle ear catarrh (glue ear) and damage to the nerve which carries the message to the brain.

The ultimate esoteric connection is a resistance to hearing what is being said as well as a desire for isolation from their world. They want to escape and find peace but it will not be found by shutting themselves away. Change is the only means of achieving inner peace but this may involve facing their fears.

In the silence, the inner word may be heard, which gives guidance to the next step on the path.

8) Tinnitus
Ringing in the ears is extremely common. It tends to be worse when there is stress and may be linked to vertigo which relates to the third eye.

The "ringing telephone" should be answered and not ignored. Once again, there is a resistance to letting go of the past and moving forward.

9) Problems of the Upper Digestive System
The digestive system, which starts at the mouth and finishes at the anus, comes partially under the control of the throat chakra and partially under the chakra in which the various sections are located. The whole process symbolises the cycle of learning through experiencing.

We ingest the experience, hopefully not biting off more than we can chew. This is then broken down by the digestive enzymes into manageable pieces and that which is useful is absorbed. This information is then assimilated for our soul growth and that which is not needed is eliminated for recycling.

The reason the digestive system connects with the throat chakra is that it is a creative process where food is taken in at one end and energy removed at another. Many of the diseases of the intestine relate to issues of control where there is conflict between "my will versus thy will".

Ingested food is under the control of the conscious mind up to the point of swallowing. After that the autonomic nervous system, which is not under the control of the conscious mind, takes over and the only control we have is to influence this nervous system through the use of the emotions.

Swallowing occurs in the area of the throat chakra and it is here that the central nervous system (my will, the will of the personality) meets the autonomic nervous system (thy will, the will of the soul).

This makes the throat chakra a very important centre for it controls the two large systems of the body, the respiratory and the digestive.

(Within the respiratory cycle there is also a small degree of control by the conscious mind ... you can hold your breath for a short period. However, the will of the soul, through the autonomic nervous system and its connection to the carotid body (see before), will naturally lead to inspiration and will therefore inevitably over-ride the will of the personality in order to maintain the life force of the individual.)

A) Mouth Ulcers

These small breaks in the lining of the mouth signify the presence of food or experiences which are creating pain within the individual. On many occasions I find that the individual is a sensitive soul who experiences life events on a deep level.

They need help to reduce their sensitivity by nurturing their own inner being and by actively expressing their feelings rather than suppressing them.

B) Chewing and Teeth

This may not be a problem but it is interesting to note how people bite into an apple for it may be symbolic of how they deal with life.

Some nibble small amounts while others bite off large pieces and wonder why they suffer indigestion! A third group chew the food many times, following advice given as a child. This group may also chew over decisions for a long time and wonder why nothing ever happens in their life.

It also fascinates me that we have one set of teeth named after wisdom. These teeth appear in the late teens and, in essence, add to the ability to grind down the food. Esoterically, one wonders if at this age that an individual is then able to ingest more knowledge and, through careful "chewing", achieve a higher level of wisdom.

The fact that so many people have their wisdom teeth removed because of small jaws, makes me question whether we are ready for the wisdom!

C) Anorexia Nervosa

This is a multi-chakra problem but there is a strong influence from the throat chakra. The condition can be found in both sexes and from late childhood onwards. There are several factors involved which include:

i) The desire to make a statement about the needs of the individual through controlling the food intake.

ii) The desire to stay a child, not to grow up and hence not to take on more responsibility. These individuals may well have grown up too fast and missed out on childhood pleasures.

iii) The desire to receive love not for what you do, but for just being yourself. Many anorexics come from families of high achievers, who combine love with success. They need to receive and give themselves unconditional love leading to enhancement of self-worth.

10) Multiple Sclerosis (M.S.)

I have spent much time in the study of diseases of the nervous system and of the muscles. The former is in some ways related to disharmony within the etheric body which is not able to cope with the incoming energies.

However, I am more and more convinced that the throat chakra is connected with M.S. and I will attempt to explain my reasons behind this conclusion. A nerve consists of a **cell body** and a long arm or **axon** which is covered with a fatty material called **myelin**. This covering not only protects the axon but also aids the conduction of the nerve impulse from the cell, along the axon to another cell body.

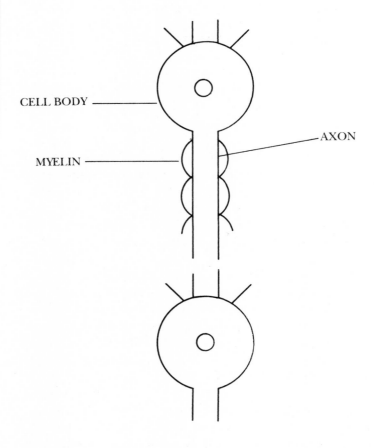

In M.S., there is initial inflammation of the myelin sheath followed by the laying down of a plaque-like material which is hard and irreversible. This material encroaches on the passage of the nerve impulse creating symptoms such as loss of sensation, loss of power, spasticity, attenuation of sensations and occasionally blindness.

Depending on the degree of plaque, in proportion to the inflammation, the disease can run a number of courses. Some people experience regular remissions with complete recovery of function, whilst others become progressively worse.

It is not clear why there are these different paths to the disease but I think we will find there are a variety of causes of M.S.

Psychospiritually, the pathology of the disease reveals an ability to accept the impulse of the soul via the cell body but an inability to transmit this into action. In other words the will to act is strong but the power is reduced, diffused and eventually dissipated (This is symbolised by the reduced passage of the impulse down the axon).

M.S. patients often have strong mental abilities with a powerful analytical mind which becomes frustrated by inactivity in relation to themselves or others. And yet there is a powerlessness to act in accordance to their own inner impulses easily swayed by the desires of others (link with solar plexus).

It is not uncommon to see the onset of symptoms occurring around the start or end of relationships with the attitude of either fierce **independence** or obvious **dependence** appearing when faced with matters requiring action.

Healing takes place when the individual learns to focus their attention and power on one step at a time without the need to manipulate or be dependent on others for this movement.

However, they also need to learn to receive without feeling in debt or vulnerable. This takes time and requires the ability to speak out from the heart concerning one's own empowerment.

Suggestions to Balance the Throat Chakra

1) Enhance your creativity through art, pottery, dance, sculpture, singing, writing, poetry, gardening and cooking.

There is no such thing as "I can't" or "I am no good at …". Every creation is as unique as the creator!

2) Choose to speak up rather than bury your feelings even though at first it may be difficult. Try writing down what you want to say first so that you can be objective and put your point across.

3) Do not assume that others will intuitively recognise your needs. Learn to ask and accept that they may say "no": on the other hand, they may say "yes"! Sometimes our outer persona does not attract help and advice. We need to show others that inside we are vulnerable and need support. Do not be too proud to ask.

4) When making a statement about yourself or your plans, do not use a phrase or tone which anticipates a negative reply.

For example:
"I'm thinking of going to some really late evening classes, what do you think?"

"You don't think I should go to evening classes do you?"

"I know it would be very inconvenient if I went to evening classes".

Use a positive statement:

"I am going to evening classes" and turn and walk away.

5) If you are a thinking person, keep a journal recording your feelings and choose to do something about those things which cause disharmony.

6) Make a list of four things you would like to do. Ask yourself if there is anything which can stop you achieving your goals. If there are major blocks are they there because you have aimed too high or are they excuses?

What makes you frightened of moving forward? Realise that you are the creator of your own future and choose to make changes now.

7) Look around your home. Are there cupboards full of items from the past which are no longer relevant to this present day? Spring-clean, whatever the season, to allow space to accommodate your future. Now spring-clean your mind, removing old emotions and thoughts.

8) The colour blue is associated with this chakra. Use it in visualisation or as an item of clothing close to the neck, to remove the blocks within this centre.

9) If you are busy with little time to spare, check that you are not running away from something which you do not wish to face.

10) Enjoy the newly created you!

The Third Eye

THE THIRD EYE

Position : Forehead
Spiritual Aspect : Self-Responsibility
Basic Need : Vision and Balance
Related Emotions : Confusion and Clarity
Endocrine Gland : Pituitary
Organs : Eyes, Lower Head, Sinuses
Colour : Indigo

Anatomy of the Pituitary Gland

This gland sits above the optic chiasma which is the meeting place of the optic nerves as they emerge from the eyes. It consists of two lobes, an anterior and a posterior, both of which secrete different hormones.

Physiology of the Pituitary Gland

This is a major gland of the body, regulating the secretion of hormones from the other glands by the release of its own hormones.

Physically, it is primarily controlled by the **hypothalamus gland** which sits above it and sends its messages via the blood stream and nervous system.

The hypothalamus receives information from different areas of the brain which are concerned with the normal functions of the body. This information covers temperature, emotions, sleep, defence mechanisms, thirst, sexual needs and hunger.

When any of these are recorded as being abnormal, messages are sent down to the pituitary gland, leading to the release of its hormones.

These hormones circulate in the blood stream until they reach their target. This may be another gland, as in the case of the thyroid, adrenal, ovaries and testes or a specific organ such as the breasts, uterus and kidneys.

The imbalance recorded in the hypothalamus is then corrected through chemical and hormonal methods; this correction is transmitted back to the hypothalamus via a "feed-back" system, which subsequently switches off the release of the hypothalamic hormones.

The hypothalamus is also one of the origins of the sympathetic nervous system which is part of the autonomic nervous system. The former is the instigator of the fight and flight response which was described under the base chakra.

Esoterically, it appears that the hypothalamus is the main gland which regulates the function of the physical body, but that it is the pituitary, with its connections to the pineal and the other glands, which is the main regulator between spirit and matter and, hence, its association with the third eye.

The Integrating Function of the Third Eye

It has been shown how the energies of the lower chakras, representing the personality, receive and merge with those of the higher chakras, representing the soul. This occurs under the guidance of the third eye. In other words, this centre reflects the unification of the soul and the personality and in essence the unification of all forms of duality. The two lobes of the pituitary gland mirror this message.

This centre also integrates the main aspects behind the creation of form. It receives from the crown the impulse which represents the will of the soul and makes a statement which expresses the intention to create in accordance with the will.

This intention is then transferred to the throat chakra which is the centre for the expression of creativity. In this way, the third eye acts as an intermediary between the will and the creative force and could be seen to represent the desire or love aspect of the soul.

Within this chakra we therefore find all three aspects of the original Source: the will, the love and the creative intelligence, which together lead to the manifestation of form which is a blend of spirit and matter.

The third eye has two arms (symbolised by the two lobes of the pituitary); one arm represents spirit and the other, matter. They are linked by a central life force which flows between the crown and the base chakras.

This triad represents the cross on which man finds himself as he aligns the power of the personality with that of the soul and starts to understand the pattern behind the Greater Plan.

Spiritual Aspect ... Self-Responsibility

The word responsibility comes from the French "spondere" which is to pledge or to promise; the full word means to promise again. Esoterically, this suggests that there is an inner commitment to manifest the impulse from the higher self into the physical body, and to receive the reaction to this manifestation as a means of soul growth.

This is symbolised by the response of the pituitary gland to higher impulses leading to release its hormones, and then to respond to the feedback from the other glands by altering this outflow.

Many individuals are very good at being responsible for other people but when it comes to their own soul needs these may be sadly lacking. Indeed, they often use this responsibility as a means of avoiding their own soul path (throat chakra).

The first priority in responsibility is to become aware of the soul's impulse and this needs practice. It appears in the form of inspiration or **intuition** and these may be ignored if the "gut feelings" of the personality shout louder.

Your intuition speaks only to you. The gut feelings or **instincts** come from previous experiences as well as from the collective consciousness. This means that they may not be specific and may therefore mislead you into following the wrong path.

To trust one's own intuition often means that you have to stand out alone and may not receive the backing of society. Many of the Great Masters have walked this path as have many men and women who have, over the centuries, significantly altered the pattern of world history.

My own way of learning to trust my intuition was by acting when I heard the same message twice. Nowadays, in most cases, I only need to be told once! Using the intuition does not guarantee an easy life but certainly makes for an interesting one, leading to an expansion in soul consciousness.

Once you know how to receive the impulse, the next question is your willingness to manifest this in the physical world. This is the conflict which may occur within the throat chakra. However, as you start to trust your intuition, the soul influence will increase and the passage of the impulse through the throat chakra will become easier.

This is the first stage in the fulfilment of the promise which you have made to yourself. The second is to respond to the feedback in a way which is going to enhance understanding and wisdom. (In the digestive system this stage can be likened to absorption and assimilation.)

It is far too easy to allow an experience to take place unwittingly whilst ignoring the underlying lesson. At other times, we become encased in the emotions of the situation or lay down belief systems which together focus on the experience rather than on the message which it carries.

Only by objectively analysing the outcome can we ever hope to move forward and this is the second stage in fulfilment of the promise.

The third eye provides us with an overview of the situation as well as receiving the impulse from above. It could be said that this eye looks in three directions. Up towards the crown and the soul impulse; down towards the base and the function of the other chakras; out through the physical eyes to the world of manifestation.

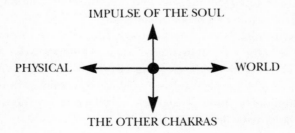

IMPULSE OF THE SOUL

PHYSICAL — WORLD

THE OTHER CHAKRAS

What we see is that which we have created, our eyes not only receiving impulses but also involved in their sending.

Related Emotions

Denial of the impulses of the soul at any level of the chakra system can lead to imbalances within the third eye. This is because that which is seen through the physical eyes, in the outer world, does not represent the vision portrayed before the third eye. Disharmony occurs, leading to dis-orientation and confusion.

The commonest cause of the problem is when the individual is working purely at the level of the personality striving to overcome issues such as insecurity, lack of confidence, the need to be needed, the feeling of being unloved, loss of control and other problems of the ego.

The only way to redress the balance is to realise that the vision of the soul is being ignored and to stop and take stock of the situation.

On many occasions, there are temporary visual problems which reflect this inner confusion. This occurs because the mind cannot cope with two different pictures and will tend to switch off one in order to rebalance the situation.

(This can also occur in a child who has a squint where, due to muscle imbalances, two pictures reach the brain. To cope with the situation, the nerve impulses from one eye are switched off, leading to a lazy eye. Unless the good eye is covered fairly quickly and the action of the lazy eye encouraged, then physical vision in that eye will be lost for ever.)

In a similar way, a compromise must be found between the two pictures: one from the soul and one from the personality, before one is switched off permanently.

If this cannot be a conscious decision, then the compromise may come in the form of mental or physical illness which helps to restore the balance. Something has to change before the onset of further turmoil and stress. This may require a period of meditation or quiet retreat and a reflection on the path which has already been walked.

Body Language

The obvious clues that someone is over-sensitive to seeing the world as it really is, are represented by the need to wear dark glasses, wear the hair over the eyes or to cover the eyes with the hands.

In essence they are also hiding themselves, believing that they cannot find harmony within the outer world. They are often highly sensitive to criticism and feel vulnerable when people come too close. They avoid visual contact, look down to the ground or over your shoulder and hope that the mask which they wear will protect them from inner scrutiny. This is strongly connected with the solar plexus and issues around self-worth and is common in the late teens where acne may also be a problem (dislike of self).

Through gentle encouragement, they need to be shown that all that they are is beautiful, and that they no longer need to hide.

They will then find that the world is far less threatening and will be able to walk with confidence rather than staring down on the ground.

Some Disease States Related to the Third Eye

1) Tension Headaches

These are related to the link between the throat chakra and the third eye and usually occur when the individual takes on more than they can handle, encouraged by the needs of the personality and refusing to listen to the intuition.

The tension may arise from the neck and shoulder areas, which suggests an attempt to "shoulder" too much responsibility and a failure to listen to their own needs.

Time is required to look within and objectively reassess the situation. This often leads to the release of burdens which were not the responsibility of the individual and allows a freedom of movement along the path.

2) Migraines

These headaches are related to changes within the blood supply to areas of the scalp and brain. Initially, there is constriction of the blood vessels, leading to sensory changes in the eyes and other parts of the body. This is then followed by dilatation of the vessels, leading to the headache, the need for darkness and possible nausea and vomiting.

There are numerous triggers for migraines including chocolate, cheese, red wine, coffee, late nights, too much sleep, stress and neck problems. All of these need to be removed if the problem is consistent.

Psychospiritually, it has been seen that such headaches are far more common in the conscientious worker who tends to keep all their problems inside. In this way there is a strong link with the type of personality who suffers with duodenal ulcers. This then links migraines partially to the solar plexus and the desire to please.

(In children, we see abdominal migraine which presents with nausea and abdominal pains. These conscientious children usually need to be reassured that they are loved for who they are and not just for what they do).

In many individuals migraines occur at weekends or at the start of holidays. This is partly due to the relaxation allowing the subconscious to express itself and partly due to the fact that this person only feels useful when at work. Rest therefore is a major stressor to the individual.

They often find it extremely difficult to be spontaneous and relaxed seen in the fact that some people find that their migraines improve with a sexual orgasm which represents complete relaxation!

Those who complain of migraines need to see where their responsibilities lie and decide not to act just to please others. They also need to learn how to act spontaneously occasionally!

3) Visual Defects
These are innumerable but the terminology can often give an indication to the possible psychospiritual disfunction:

A) Short-sightedness
This commonly relates to a state of mind as well as a state of vision. There is a tendency to become too involved in present day details with a fear of looking into the future.

B) Long-sightedness

This may relate to those who live in the past and the future and avoid the present. They have a fear of facing that which is happening right in front of their eyes. They should be shown that by facing up to the truth they can also be moved through their own fears.

C) Glaucoma

This is a condition where the pressure of the fluid within the eyes is increased, leading to strain upon the optic nerve and possible blindness.

The initial visual loss is in the periphery, leading to "tunnel-vision". Psychospiritually, these people often appear to have tunnel-vision in their dealings with the rest of the world. They can be hard and intolerant of the needs of others, often built upon many years of personal suffering.

I remember a woman with blindness caused by glaucoma having to learn to accept help from others which she had previously refused. In this way she come to love herself and her fellow man.

D) Cataracts

This disease affects the lens of the eye. This translucent structure allows light to pass through it from the outside onto the sensitive retina which records chemically and neurologically that which has been seen.

The lens changes its shape in order to accommodate the distance from the object viewed to the eye.

When a cataract is formed the lens has become hard and opaque, preventing light from entering the eye.

Psychospiritually, it represents a feeling of "sameness" about life, with the fear that there may not be the heights of joy again and within this a dark vision of the future.

With all the visual disturbances, darkness may occur. However, within the void, a small light can often be seen which was not noticed before. This light represents the light of the soul.

E) Astigmatism

This condition occurs when the surfaces of the two eyes are not symmetrical. It is a congenital problem and suggests that the individual is here to learn to find balance through the use of their third eye which is linked with intuition.

F) Floaters

These little black dots seen within the visual field are said medically to be due to the breakdown of the fluid within the eye.

In esoteric terms, the eye is related to the liver and the floaters become more noticeable when there are disturbances in the energy flow of this organ caused by such emotions as anger, resentment and frustration.

One is not only seeing "red" but even "black". Resolve the anger and the floaters will recede.

4) Catarrh and Sinus Problems

The normal secretions of the nose are formed to protect the respiratory passages from pollutants. They are produced in excess, as catarrh, during infections as well as in response to certain food substances or irritants to which the nose and sinuses have become hypersensitive.

Psychospiritually, the hypersensitivity relates back to the heart chakra and an overactive immune system which needs to be balanced.

However, there are also other connections which include:

A) A post nasal drip occurs when catarrh runs down the back of the throat causing the individual to swallow frequently, to cough or to feel a lump in the throat.

Esoterically, this is related to tears which have not been shed; these can be tears of frustration as well as tears of grief.

B) Sinusitis

There are four sinuses or air spaces found within the face which are used to amplify the resonance of the voice and to lighten the skull.

The most commonly affected, by infection or allergy, are the maxillary (within the cheeks) and the frontal (across the forehead).

Esoterically, maxillary sinusitis relates to the throat chakra and feelings of frustration and anger caused by an inability to express oneself. Frontal sinusitis relates to the third eye and expresses confusion and inner tears as the path forward is not clear.

The sinuses can be cleared by dealing with the emotions as well as by removing the irritants from the environment.

Suggestions to Balance the Third Eye

1) Learn to use the intuition. It is probably the first thought which comes into the mind; the second is the gut instinct.

2) Sit and meditate or find a quiet place where you can recall the experiences of the day, retaining those which are useful and discarding the rest.

3) Learn to look beyond the situation. See things from the level of the higher self rather than from the ego.

4) If there is confusion, understand that it is the outer picture which needs to change, not the one from within.

5) Ask yourself if you are keeping the promises which you made to your Creator, ie. allowing the full potential of your inner being to be seen.

6) Look back at your life and check whether you are learning through your mistakes or just repeating the pattern.

Choose to change.

7) The colour connected with this chakra is indigo. It is seen in the depth of an ocean and the vastness of the sky at night. It denotes that there is no limit to your creativity and that the only thing which limits you, is you. Use this colour to widen your horizons.

8) See the world as a place of boundless possibilities where there is space for work and play.

Chapter 13

The Crown Chakra

THE CROWN CHAKRA

Position : Top of Head
Spiritual Aspect : Self-Consciousness
Basic Need : Acceptance
Related Emotions : Despair and Peace
Endocrine gland : Pineal
Associated Organs : Brain
Colour : Violet/Purple

Anatomy of the Pineal Gland

This pea-sized gland arises from the roof of the third ventricle of the brain. It is superior and posterior to both the hypothalamus and pituitary glands. It has several nerve endings but it is not entirely clear as to their origin or target.

Physiology of the Pineal Gland

Until recently little was known about this gland except that in later life it becomes calcified. This information was previously used as a form of diagnosis. For when there is a space-occupying lesion, such as a tumour or blood clot within the brain, the gland is pushed over to one side and this can be seen on X-ray. Modern scans, however, have rendered this form of diagnosis redundant.

In the past few years increasing interest has been shown in trying to understand the connection between this gland and the rest of the body.

The French philosopher, Descartes (1596–1650), described the pineal gland as the seat of the soul. In animals, the gland is known to be strongly linked with the function of the sex

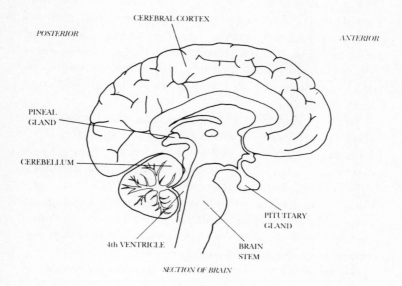

CEREBRAL CORTEX

POSTERIOR

ANTERIOR

PINEAL
GLAND

CEREBELLUM

PITUITARY
GLAND

4th VENTRICLE

BRAIN
STEM

SECTION OF BRAIN

glands, leading to suppression of sexual function in the winter months and release of sex hormones in the summer months.

Man's reproductive desires do not follow the seasons but it has been speculated that the pineal has a connection with the regulation of rhythms within the body, especially those involved with hormone release.

The main hormone produced by this gland is **melatonin**. This is not the exclusive site of its production for it is now being found in many other parts of the body.

The manufacture of this hormone is increased during the dark and decreases during the light. It has therefore been implicated in problems such as jet-lag and S.A.D. (seasonal affected disorder). Its release is also thought to be related to heat although the exact connection is not clear.

Melatonin is synthesized from the essential amino acid **tryptophan** which then forms **serotonin** and finally melatonin. Tryptophan has been used for many years to relieve depression and insomnia.

Serotonin is a neurotransmitter within the brain, sending

messages from one area to another. Medical studies have revealed that disturbances of the serotonin level, both high and low, are seen in patients with Parkinson's disease and schizophrenia. It is not clear whether this is cause or effect although it may well be that research will find that several diseases exist under the one heading, each relating to different levels of serotonin.

To recap: it is known that the pineal gland is light, and probably heat, sensitive and appears to act as a regulating force both for hormonal release as well as for the release of several neurotransmitters involved in sending messages within the brain.

Esoterically, I believe that the fact that melatonin is produced in the dark, ie. at night or during meditation, suggests that it is during this time that the impulses from the soul enter the right brain through the crown chakra and start their passage through the nervous system until manifestation.

It is during winter that all of nature becomes surrounded by darkness. However, the seed of life contained within the soul continues to shine. It is at this time that we reflect on our path and allow new inspiration to enter our consciousness.

I believe that those who suffer with the depression of S.A.D. are unable to find their inner light and rely on the artificial lights of the outside world.

Another finding concerning the pineal gland, is that it appears to be affected by electro-magnetic fields and in some way helps to improve our sense of direction. This concept was revealed in two experiments.

One involved a group of people who were lost on Exmoor in Devon, England, who fell and knocked their heads; subsequent skull X-rays showed, as an incidental finding, that they had calcified pineal glands. In comparison, a similar group of patients also with head injuries but who had not been lost, were X-rayed. In this group the gland had not calcified.

The hypothesis suggests that a non-calcified pineal gland allows us to connect with magnetic energies leading to a good sense of direction.

The other experiment used small aquatic animals which also have melatonin within their nervous system. These were placed within a large magnetic shield and taken from the Pacific Ocean to the Atlantic. When they were released into the water, still within the shield, they swam round and round in circles. Removal of the shield saw them turn in the direction of the Pacific and start to swim home.

Esoterically, I believe that these two examples suggest that the pineal gland is sensitive not only to the electro-magnetic force of the earth's core but also to that of our inner sun or soul.

I watch with interest as the information concerning this gland increases and believe that many more related hormones will be discovered with connections throughout the body, especially to other glands and to the autonomic nervous system.

Spiritual Aspect ... Self-Consciousness

The crown chakra connects with the will aspect of the Creator (the Light who made all life) through the "thread of con-sciousness", providing us with the "will-to-be" without condi-tions or expectations. The centre is most active during infancy as this energy becomes embedded within the physical body. (Indeed it is thought that the closure of the anterior fontanelle of the skull between 12 and 18 months of life reflects the com-pletion of this process.)

During the remaining years of our life, and for most lifetimes on this planet, we strive to strengthen the link between our-selves and our Creator through the development of self-consciousness.

It is only when our soul is fully incarnate within the physical body and is expressed through the base chakra that we reach full understanding (under-stand) of our place in the Greater Plan.

This energy can then be lifted to the crown and our soul's vibration will merge with that of the Creator, bringing ultimate peace. Such highly enlightened beings then express the will of the Creator and not that of the individual soul.

As with the heart chakra, this centre is not highly developed in the majority of the population. However, the consciousness of man is ever-expanding due to pressures from the higher planes of existence and this is expressed in the increasing interest in esoteric matters.

When the spiritual link is poor, or when the energy from the crown chakra is resisted, the individual may lose their "will-to-live" which is one of the symptoms of depression.

Self-consciousness is to know and love yourself in all your aspects: mind, body and spirit and within this to allow the three to become one.

Body Language

Total despair is revealed when someone places their hands over the top of their head. They feel that they have no connection with life and are lost. In most cases, they cannot receive the messages from their higher self due to their own desperation. They need unconditional and loving guidance to help them once again receive the light.

Many religions require their followers to cover the top of the head, revealing their understanding of the sacredness of this centre.

Some Disease States Related to the Crown Chakra

1) Depression

In reactive depression, there is loss of direction and purpose in life. This often occurs after the death of a partner, loss of a job, separation of a marriage or is related to any other event which will precipitate change. It can occur during any stage of the grief process but particularly at a time of confusion and disorientation.

Esoterically, the link with the "will-to-be" is poor and the eyes are turned away from the light. However, as stated previously, it is in the darkness that the light shines brightest and, with or without the help of the various therapies to lift the depression, there comes a time when the individual reaches the limit of their despair and there is only one way to go, and that is up. Every ocean has an ocean bed; every emotion reaches the bottom at some point and recovery occurs.

How much easier it would be to see the light on the way down rather than having to go all the way to the bottom. Some choose not to continue their life, but premature death leaves an incarnation unfinished and the soul must return to complete its contract.

There are others who are prone to depression for most of their lives. The blame is often placed at the door of their childhood and yet other children in similar situations do not suffer to such a degree.

I believe that within these individuals the "will-to-be" is poorly received at the crown chakra and there is resistance to being here on earth, which may be related to past life experiences.

Through help and encouragement, they need to find not only a purpose for life but a will to live. Esoterically, we cannot keep blaming the world for the conditions in which we find ourselves, for it is my belief that we choose these situations for our own soul growth.

Looking beyond the experiences helps one to move forward and this can only happen when we are willing to release all that is no longer valid in our life. Holding on to anger, despair, resentment, etc. will always create a heavy burden and does not change the past. We are the creators of our future; choose wisely that which you wish to represent this time.

2) Parkinson's Disease
This disease represents a deficiency in the neurotransmitter **dopamine** leading to restriction of voluntary movement, tremor and rigidity. These patients lose facial expression and the natural swing of the arms when walking. There is often an accompanying depression although the lack of facial expression frequently masks a sense of humour.

There are known to be several causative factors for the illness although most cases are said to be idiopathic (cause unknown).

Within the area of voluntary movement, the basic problem is one of initiating activity, leading to a reliance on gravity when getting out of a chair or moving forward from the position of standstill. (Gravity is the major energy influencing the base chakra.)

This lack of motivation is a feature of the mind, often apparent before the onset of the disease. I find that many of these individuals have been poorly self-motivated and are commonly reliant on a strong partner or family who does everything for them. Unfortunately, the slowness which accompanies the disease leads to the temptation by others to speed up any event, by taking over basic tasks. This should be discouraged where possible.

Esoterically, this disease represents a closed crown chakra with little true self-consciousness, and a wide open base chakra representing reliance on the external world for security.

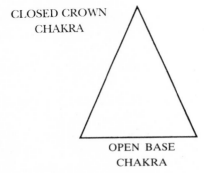

CLOSED CROWN
CHAKRA

OPEN BASE
CHAKRA

Once the disease has manifest, it is difficult to motivate change within the patterns of a lifetime but this should be encouraged where possible. I hope that through greater understanding of spiritual man we may be able to prevent the onset of this disease. However, prevention is very difficult to measure as lack of symptoms is the hallmark of success!

3) Schizophrenia

This is a disease where there are major thought disturbances creating difficulties for the individual to live within the rational world. These disturbances include hearing voices, paranoia, tangential thinking, word associations and visual illusions. (Many of these features are also seen in those with highly developed psychic abilities; the only difference is that the latter hopefully know the difference between reality and illusion.)

Medically, it is thought that there is a chemical defect within the brain which may be associated with a particular type of environmental upbringing.

Esoterically, the etheric body of the crown chakra is over-sensitive, acting as antennae to receive messages not only from the higher self but also from the surrounding environment, including those from the collective consciousness.

The crown chakra is far too open and the individual is unable to deal rationally with the impulses he receives. I believe that the main defect is in the connection between the right intuitive and left logical brain.

I have found that many schizophrenic patients have well developed thought-processes from an early age but find themselves in a family where free creative expression is repressed due to strict standards and high expectations. These factors lead to tight boundaries being created on a young mind, leading to an obsessive nature often seen in hobbies where extreme fastidiousness is required, eg. stamp collecting.

At the time of puberty, when there is a natural need to break free of family restrictions, this creativity appears to be restricted and the only way out is through the top of the head.

Esoterically, there is a tightly closed base chakra allowing poor grounding on the earth due to basic insecurity and a wide open crown chakra.

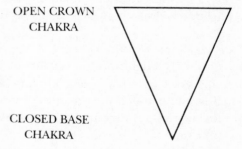

OPEN CROWN
CHAKRA

CLOSED BASE
CHAKRA

If the individual can be reached, they should be encouraged to reduce any spiritual or intellectual activities and to become more involved in everyday tasks, especially those which are connected with the earth, eg. gardening and farming. This will help to ground their impulses whilst still enhancing the freedom of creative expression.

4) Epilepsy

There are two main types of epilepsy: grand mal and petit mal (absences). They are both related to electrical disturbances within the brain. In the former there is a full-blown fit with loss of consciousness and shaking whilst in petit mal there are periods of blankness.

Both can occur without any known cause although there may be a family history of the disease. Grand mal is often seen after trauma to the head, after birth trauma and is commonly triggered by emotional stress.

The fits of petit mal, which are more common in children, can be brought on by flashing lights which create an interface between light and dark. These include the lights used to produce television pictures, strobe lighting, the light seen through the steps of an escalator, the sun flashing through passing trees when in a car or train and the dimmed light of twilight.

Many individuals with petit mal are extremely sensitive to atmospheric changes and can detect the approach of a storm while it is still some miles away. They also pick up the emotional atmosphere of others in a room, via the solar plexus, and use the fit as a means of escaping from the situation. Many adults use the same ploy by day-dreaming when things become too difficult!

Whatever the cause or type of epilepsy, I believe that psychospiritually there is a defect in the stability of the link between matter and spirit and that, during a fit, the life force of the individual is split between the energies of this three-dimensional world and those of four dimensions found within the next plane of existence.

The energies in the base chakra are poorly connected to the earth at this time and this shift of energies can be likened to the state of semi-consciousness which occurs just prior to sleep.

Using grounding exercises, as well as accepting the desire to be on this earth, helps to alleviate the symptoms.

5) Senile Dementia

In this illness there is atrophy or thinning of the cerebral cortex, the outer layer of the brain.

It is characterised by memory loss, emotional instability, insomnia, loss of reason and judgement, delusions and often loss of personal integrity. In many cases the individuals become almost childlike and require constant vigilance and guidance.

Psychospiritually, it is seen that many of these people have been somewhat pragmatic in their lives, relying on logic rather than feelings, which were suppressed; they need to be in control either emotionally or physically.

It appears that the dementia brings to the surface the child within, plus all the buried feelings, rebalancing the situation which for too long has been held in one extreme and allows them to leave this earth with much more ease.

Some Suggestions to Balance the Crown Chakra

1) Sit or lie in a comfortable position for meditation. Remove shoes and loosen all tight clothing. Make sure that your back and head are well supported and that your arms and legs are not crossed. Rest your hands comfortably.

Take three deep breaths letting go of stresses on each out-breath. Now proceed to relax your body by releasing any tension from your muscles starting in the feet and working up to the scalp. Let the tension go into the ground and leave your body heavy, relaxed and at peace.

Next, take yourself to your safe-place; a place you may know or only dream about. Here, there is utter peace and tranquillity. Become aware of your surroundings using your inner eyes, ears, nose and touch.

When you feel ready to move on, see above an energy which represents your higher self; it may take a form, be represented by colour or be abstract.

Allow the energies of your crown chakra to rise up and merge with this form. Feel your mind clear as the will of your higher self takes over from the thoughts of the day and fills it with peace.

Now bring that energy down through the crown chakra and

down to the base chakra, allowing it to enter every cell of the body, replacing disharmony with peace.

When the energy reaches the base chakra, let it pass out through the feet deep into the ground where it links with the will of mother earth.

See these two energies merge and then rise together up through the base to the crown and up to the higher self again. Continue to allow the energies to circle between the higher self and mother earth with your body as the receiver of these energies. You are now totally in the present and in the "presence" of your Creator.

Enjoy this feeling for a few moments.

When you are ready, bring the energy down from the higher self to the crown and up from mother earth to the base and be at peace. Close each chakra in turn, starting at the crown; this can be likened to watching a flower close.

When they are all closed, surround yourself with a white or golden light so that you can continue the day's activities.

Use this exercise whenever you feel that you have lost your way or when you feel disconnected from your Source.

2) The colours violet or purple can be used as a means of balancing the chakra either in the clothes which are worn or during visualisation.

3) Choose to find peace and joy in your life and to give yourself 10 minutes every day just to sit quietly and replenish your own energies.

4) Be at peace with yourself and with the world.

Summary of the Upper Three Chakras

The Heart Chakra is the centre for the reception of the love of the soul and, through the soul, links with the Love of the Creator.

The Throat Chakra is the centre for the reception of the mind of the soul and, through the soul, links with the Mind of the Creator.

The Crown Chakra is the centre which is receptive to the will of the soul and, through the soul, links with the Will of the Creator.

Chapter 14

Other Psychospiritual Links with Disease

Sides of the Body

The **right side of the body** represents the **masculine** side of one's character, relating to assertiveness, activity, expressiveness, logical thinking and strength.

The **left side of the body** represents the **feminine** side and relates to sensitivity, passivity, receptivity, intuition, and nurturing.

They also reflect personal and emotional associations, with the right side symbolising the father and other men and the left side the mother and other women.

During the development of our masculine and feminine aspects, leading to their eventual interaction, there are times when areas of emotional disharmony will manifest within the physical body.

I see many people whose symptoms always appear on the one side signifying that there is an important message to be learnt in relation to this area.

For example:

1) Jenny presented with stiffness and pain in her right elbow, shoulder and great toe which caused her great difficulty when driving her car.

On further questioning it became apparent that much of her life was spent in the car, ferrying children to school, visiting aged parents and in-laws, and shopping for neighbours.

When asked how she felt about these jobs, she responded

with a definite "resentful" and immediately felt guilty for expressing this emotion.

The right side of her body is her expressive side and the joints, which represent movement, are blocked by feelings which are not being expressed.

If this persists, the joints will become so stiff that she will no longer be able to drive and the physical body will solve the problem without the need for verbal expression, ie. she will not be able to be general chauffeuse for all concerned.

However, such stiffness may also restrict other activities which she enjoys and may lead to irreversible damage.

With counselling, she was able to say "No" when appropriate and to divide her time more equally between that spent on the needs of others and that required for herself.

2) I am asked to see a boy who has pain in his lower back. On examination, I find that his left hip is raised higher than his right and that this has created an imbalance in the muscle tensions of the back leading to a mild scoliosis (twist of the spine).

On further questioning, I find him to be an extremely talented young artist who through his art can express his sensitivity and the way he sees the world.

However, his family disapprove of the time spent on this talent and are pressing him to achieve academically at school. He feels torn (twisted) between his desire to express his creativity and his desire to please his parents.

Six months previously he had laid down his brushes and buried his head in his books.

This young man had found that when his sensitive creativity touched the earth it was not accepted and, in order to restore harmony on one level, he had lifted his left foot marginally off the ground thereby lifting the hip. This had however created the pain in the lower back due to the muscle tension.

We talked about his love of painting and I agreed to see him next time with one of his parents. Whilst we discussed the need to see an osteopath, I also brought up the question of his art. As a family they eventually reached a compromise, allowing him an hour a day for art as long as he had finished his homework.

Locked into the body may be many years and lifetimes of pain, disappointment, hurt and anger. By understanding the message in terms of masculinity and femininity, the key to releasing these emotions is far easier to find.

JOINTS

Joints are the physical structures involved with movement and vary in their range of activity, from the joints between the skull bones which have practically no movement, to the wrist which can turn in many directions.

Each joint moves the individual through different aspects of life; disease in a joint can represent blockage of the energy flow relating to this aspect.

For example:
The Shoulder represents ... carrying and lifting.

Disharmony relates to being overburdened by the problems of others and the need to unload for the sake of all concerned.

The Elbow represents ... acceptance.

Disharmony relates to the desire to push things or people away.

There is a need to accept what is offered whilst confidently remaining in control.

The Wrist represents ... creative freedom.

Disharmony relates to a feeling of restriction. There is a need to acknowledge this feeling and work towards release.

The Fingers represent ... fine adjustments to life.

Disharmony relates to becoming hampered by detail or becoming insensitive to the delicate balance of nature.

There is a need to become flexible and hence lighten the movement of the fingers.

Pointing of the index finger expresses a desire to judge or blame others rather than looking for a cause within oneself.

The Hip represents ... stability in movement.

Disharmony relates to the inability to move forward confidently whether due to fear or feelings of insecurity.

There is a need to become more self-assured and hence more securely linked with the higher self in all movement.

The Knee represents ... humility and pride.

Disharmony relates to the inability to release one's pride and to be humble. Many people are **too** humble and need to get up off their knees in order to regain self-respect.

The Ankle represents ... freedom of movement.

Disharmony relates to a feeling of restriction in the direction one wants to take, eg. to take a new job or to move home.

Expression of the desire often leads to new mobility.

The Toes represent ... fine adjustments to forward movement.

Disharmony relates to becoming hampered by worries of the future or the feeling of being held back by details.

When the higher mind is working with the personality each step forward can be taken in the knowledge that there is no wrong step along the path.

Gout of the great toe usually symbolises frustration and anger which is preventing forward movement (we move off from this toe).

Bunions of the great toe, often due to shoe fashions, represent someone who would rather follow others than their own path.

THE SPINE

The vertebral column gives support to the spinal cord which carries nerve impulses to and from the brain. In man, it also offers support to our vertical position.

The psychospiritual meaning of disharmony in the spine will depend on the area affected:

a) **Lumbar spine** (lower back) reflects a feeling that the burdens have become too great and there is often underlying resentment that nobody else is there to help.

b) **Thoracic spine** (chest area) reflects lack of space for expression of hurt and anger.

c) **Cervical spine** (neck) reflects a lack of flexibility due to an inability or fear of looking in all directions.

A **slipped disc** anywhere, represents a feeling of being unsupported and unable to cope.

THE SKIN

The skin is our main interface with the outside world and represents "me as an individual" in relation to the rest of society. It reflects and communicates one's inner feelings towards this environment. Natural expression of feelings is often a problem for those with skin disorders.

There are various ways in which disharmony can manifest within the skin:

A) Thickening of the skin

This occurs over areas which are prone not only to physical but also mental trauma and acts as a protective mechanism.

Nothing seems to affect someone with a "thick skin". However, this protective covering has usually been developed over a period of time, often in response to early emotional pain which was suppressed due to an unfriendly environment. From then on there is a strict policy that nothing will hurt them again and such individuals find it difficult to trust.

Those who suffer with "prickly heat", where sweat builds up behind a non-porous skin, also present with this protective barrier.

In Chinese medicine, the skin relates to the lung meridian and through this, esoterically, is linked to the throat chakra –

the centre of self-expression. Grief, hurt and pain are the commonest emotions contained behind the skin.

Unfortunately, not only does it keep pain out, it also keeps pain in. Others are unable to come close and offer love and support leaving the individual feeling isolated and unable to interact fully with society.

In **Reflexology** it is seen that the hardened areas on the soles of the feet (callouses) relate to the areas in the body where the individual feels he/she needs protection.

Psoriasis is a condition where there is a thickening of the epidermis, usually occurring on the more exposed surfaces of the body, ie. areas more vulnerable to trauma (emotional or physical). Psoriasis is most prevalent at times of stress and improves with ultraviolet light which may be natural (the sun) or artificial.

Psychospiritually, I usually find that patients with psoriasis initially appear defensive with a need to be in control of the consultation. However, as time goes on, I meet a very sensitive and vulnerable inner child who needs nurturing and encouragement to find and express themselves rather than hide away from life by laying down further layers of skin as a means of protection.

Some people develop psoriasis over the occipital bone which is found at the base of the skull. This area forms an important link between the throat chakra and the third eye and represents an unwillingness to express what is seen before their own eyes.

B) Dermatitis

This condition represents inflammation of the skin whether due to chemicals, foods, trauma or stress. It is related to disharmony of the immune response which mainly involves the solar plexus and heart chakras.

Eczema is a specific form of dermatitis often found in association with asthma and hay fever. The presenting symptoms are a red, irritating, scaly rash which may later become weepy or infected. The surfaces involved are usually those hidden from view such as inside the elbow or behind the knee. This

reflects the hiding of emotions and the sensitivity of the individual.

Although each part of this formula will be discussed below,
eczema represents a hypersensitivity to something within the
environment, physical or emotional, which in the case of the
emotions is being suppressed for fear of upsetting others.

Red or burning skin reflects suppressed anger and frustration
and the need to express these feelings more openly.

Itching always reflects irritation with something or someone
but with an inability to escape from the situation.

Something has "got under the skin" and the body is attempting to force this irritation out onto the surface so that it can be
seen and dealt with.

Weeping of the skin often reveals unresolved inner tears and
that the body is aiding in their release.

C) Boils occur when there is an infection of the sebaceous
glands (which supply sebum to the skin) and reflect something
which has been festering for some time and needs to "come to
a head". Symbolically, it is important to get to the root of the
real problem rather just deal with the superficial effects (the
pus).

A "blind" boil reflects the inability to let go of the past or to
express deep emotions, often to the detriment of the individual.

D) Acne is caused by excessive secretions from the sebaceous
glands and is normally associated with the male hormones.

It is common in the teens and early twenties when an individual is developing their sense of sexual identity. But acne can
occur at any age when there is an imbalance between the masculine and feminine aspects of the person, leading to lack of
confidence and poor self-love.

In women, it is commonly seen when excessive amounts of
the male hormones are being released which can represent
suppression of the feminine side.

E) Acne Rosacea is a condition more commonly found in
women where there is an imbalance in the nerve control of the

blood vessels, leading to their dilatation with redness of the cheeks and nose as well as small spots or pimples.

There are certain triggers which cause this imbalance which include alcohol, smoking, dairy products, spices and, most commonly, suppressed anger and indignation.

These people are often pleasers who do not want to upset or hurt others but who feel angry that their needs are not being heard.

They need to learn to speak out and not to fear the consequences.

F) Warts and Verrucas are caused by a virus invading the skin. These are common at times of self-searching when those parts of our being which are less lovable come to the surface. It really is important to love ourselves "warts and all".

Alopecia

This is a condition where there is loss of hair, mainly from the head but also from other sites. There is commonly a past history of shock which literally "shook the roots" of the person's being, and the shock and subsequent grief remained within the hair bed preventing further growth.

The scalp hair has always been seen as a sign of strength, which is probably because it covers the crown chakra. In healing, the grief needs to be dealt with while encouragement is given to build inner strength and security.

Chapter 15

The Way Forward

Over the centuries there have been many changes within the pattern of healing. Modern medicine only came into existence at the end of the last century, prior to which those medicines which are now called "alternative" were then in vogue.

At present, there is a swing back to the more natural forms of healing as the reliance on synthetic drugs has failed to live up to expectations. There is no "pill for every ill" and, despite the most sophisticated technology, people are still becoming ill and dying.

Maybe it is time we stopped trying to devise another form of medicine and started to look at the whole process of disease and its relationship to health.

To do this we must break down the barriers which exist between religion, philosophy, psychology and medicine and realise that they each represent only part of the whole picture. Until they all unite under a common banner they will continue to provide a poor service to any who seek their help.

To be healthy is to be whole and this occurs through the unification of the mind, the body and the spirit. This goal is reached via a path upon which we find situations which provide us with opportunities to experience all aspects of life contained within a human existence.

However, we are not to be blinded by the experience but should look beyond and see the lessons which are revealed. Through these we learn to accept all parts of ourselves and eventually to love them. This is the way to the expansion of soul consciousness and to ultimate wholeness.

Disease is a signpost along the path which signals a time for change. It appears initially as disharmony within the mind and if this does not bring about transformation then it manifests in the body as physical disease.

The change which takes place may lead to remission of the symptoms, a chronic illness or death. All are part of the soul's path. There is no point in someone staying on the earth if their work here is finished. In death, the soul simply moves to a new plane of existence.

Whatever happens to an individual in their life is not a coincidence. We are given freewill to respond to the experiences offered but if the soul is determined to move the individual forward then this will happen.

The role of preventive medicine must also change, for success cannot be measured on whether the patient lives or dies. This is not in the hands of the carer.

So where does this leave the healing arts?

I believe that it is time for three things to happen:

1) All therapists, whether orthodox or complementary, should consider the whole person: mind, body and spirit and, after "first aid" treatment, apply their healing art to encompass as much as possible of the total being.

2) Recognition should be given to the importance of allowing a patient to resume responsibility for their own health. They can then choose to receive the most appropriate treatment and advice available to help them through this period of change.

3) All therapists must recognise that they are acting as a mirror for the patient to see their true self. If the mirror is dirty then the picture will be obscured. It is therefore important that all those practising within the caring professions work towards putting their own house in order so as to provide as clear a reflection as possible.

Any therapy is only as good as the therapist.

Times are changing fast and barriers are being removed all over the world. But the greatest barriers are those still present within our minds.

Last week, Molly came to see me with cancer of the breast. The original lump had appeared shortly after she had felt a stabbing pain in her chest. The cancer had been removed but now she had developed a secondary in the same breast which on examination appeared as a hard, hot lump distorting the contours of the body.

We talked about diet, general health and orthodox treatments. I then asked whether there was anything in the past couple of years which she could connect with the cancer.

She willingly volunteered this information. Fourteen months ago she had gone to stay with her daughter and grandchildren. She loved her daughter and had worked hard to give her the life that she herself would have wanted. During the stay, her daughter asked Molly not to criticise her children and said that she would bring them up in her own way.

Molly said that this comment went right through her "like a stabbing knife". She could not believe that her daughter could be so thoughtless after all she had done for her. She was deeply hurt and since the event had not spoken or written to her daughter. Six months later the first cancer had appeared. The daughter had pleaded with her mother to return her calls or to write, but to no avail. She did not know that Molly had been in hospital as her father had been forbidden to pass on this information.

Molly concluded by saying that she knew that the cancer was connected to her hurt. I asked her what her daughter had to do to get back into her favour. "Nothing" she replied. "You're punishing her, aren't you?" I said. "Yes" she answered with defiance.

Her breast lump was as firm as she was in her attitude towards her daughter. The heat was coming from her anger. She had nurtured this child at her breast and now the child had rejected her. The anger and hurt were fixed within the breast tissue.

"In the end the person who is being punished is yourself", I said. "I know", she replied with a sigh, and reverted to asking what forms of therapy were available for cancer.

Molly had the courage to be honest for which I was full of admiration because this is rare. But despite this, she was not willing to release her emotional hold over her daughter and to offer the hand of forgiveness, even though it would lead to further pain and suffering and probable death.

Disease is a period of transition. For true healing to occur it is the attitude of the mind which must be transformed. Here is an opportunity to throw out the old records and to select something new to play.

All this requires courage and can only come when each individual learns to love themself unconditionally.

We are on our paths alone and only here will we find our inner truth. Now is the time to pass through the door of transformation and to walk towards the light of the soul bearing its gifts of peace, joy and wholeness.

For information on future workshops please write to the author via her publisher.

BIBLIOGRAPHY

Esoteric Healing, Alice Bailey; The Lucis Press

Radionics & the Subtle Anatomy of Man, David Tansley; The C.W. Daniel Co. Ltd

Cutting the Ties that Bind, Phyllis Krystal; Element Books

You Can Heal Your Life, Louise Hay; Eden Grove Editions

You Can Fight for Your Life, Laurence Le Shan; Thorson Publishing Group

Quantum Healing, Deepak Chopra; Bantam Books

Love, Medicine and Miracles, Bernie Siegel; Harper & Row Ltd

Index